About the Author

Elizabeth Danciger was born in Memphis, Tennessee. She has lived in Europe since early childhood, and has spent the greater part of her life in England. Before training as a Homoeopath, she was an artist and art historian, and a teacher of both. The study of history and the history of ideas has always been one of her main concerns. She is a practising homoeopath with her practice in London, and is also a teacher of Homoeopathy and the history of medicine.

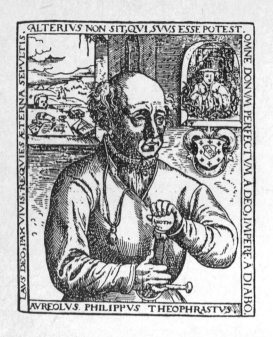

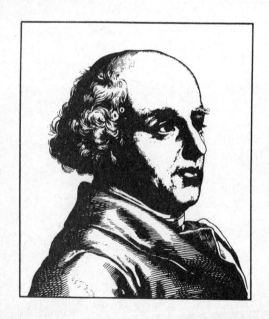

HOMEOPATHY
FROM ALCHEMY
TO MEDICINE

Elizabeth Danciger

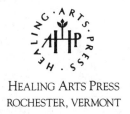

HEALING ARTS PRESS
ROCHESTER, VERMONT

Dedicated
to
my
mother and father,
Leila and Jacob,
and
to
my
homoeopathic teacher,
John Da Monte

Healing Arts Press
One Park Street
Rochester, Vermont 05767

LIBRARY OF CONGRESS CATALOGING-IN-
PUBLICATION DATA

Danciger, Elizabeth
  Homeopathy : from alchemy to medicine
by Elizabeth Danciger.
    p.   cm.
  Bibliography: p.
  Includes index.
  ISBN 0-89281-290-7
  1. Homeopathy   I. Title
RX71.D36 1988   88-36504
615.5'32'09--dc19   CIP

Printed and bound in the United States

10 9 8 7 6 5 4 3 2 1

Healing Arts Press is a division of Inner Traditions
International, Ltd.

Distributed to the book trade in the United States by Harper and
    Row Publishers, Inc.
Distributed to the book trade in Canada by Book Center, Inc.,
    Montreal, Quebec
Distributed to the health food trade in Canada by Alive Books,
    Toronto and Vancouver

Contents

Preface vi
1 Hahnemann and Homoeopathy 1
2 Paracelsus 11
3 The Iatrochemists and the Scientific Revolution 33
4 The Rosicrucian Element 49
5 Medicine and the Enlightenment 69
6 Hahnemann 83
Index 105

Preface

This book will hopefully fulfill the present need to give some background to the four centuries of medical, scientific and philosophical history in Europe leading to the period in which Homoeopathy was formulated as a medical science. The subject is a vast one. I have attempted to remain economic in ideas so that what I believe to be a coherent evolution of events and ideas can be discerned. One could write volumes about each of the many areas touched upon, and yet that was not fully relevant here.

In my days of training as a Homoeopathic practitioner, I was obsessed with finding the roots of the medicine I was studying. Thus began a journey into many areas of history I had not yet encountered. I learned a myriad of things which led me to yet other avenues of discovery, all of which inspired me as I worked at acquiring the tools for the practice of Homoeopathy. Certainly not everyone is concerned with history, but I have found that by unravelling the past, the present always takes on a new and clearer dimension.

Thus I hope this journey will also be of interest to the reader, inspiring perhaps further study or reading, or just an awareness of some of the roots of a fascinating and certainly very important method of cure, becoming more and more widely appreciated and needed today.

I would very much like to express my many thanks to two great scholars, whom we have sadly lost in the last few years, for their support and assistance in my years of research, which have since been synthesized into this book. Namely, to Frances Yates, late Fellow of the Warburg Institute, and Walter Pagel, one of the leading Paracelsian scholars of our century. Without their help and pointers along the way I'd have had a far harder task indeed in finding my material and keeping on the right track of discovery. I would also like to express my thanks to many friends and relatives who have been supportive and very helpful during the preparation of this book, and to the various people in particular for their assistance in the editorial work and preparation of the manuscript. Leila Ward in particular for her untiring assistance, as well as David Haight and Jack Meyers, and my colleagues, Rima Handley, and Francis Treuhertz, for being such thoughtful and helpful readers of the manuscript in preparation.

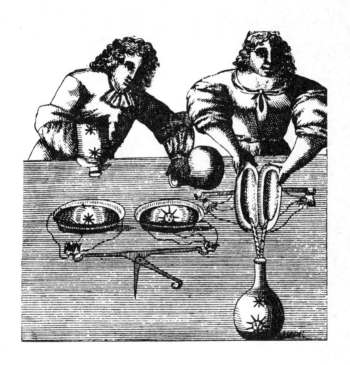

1 Hahnemann and Homoeopathy

The Physician's first duty is to enquire into the whole condition of the patient – the cause of the disease, his mode of life, the nature of his mind, the tone and character of his sentiments, his physical constitution, and especially the symptoms of his disease.

Samuel Hahnemann

'Pathos', the ancient Greek word for 'suffering', is a vital component of Homoios-pathos, meaning 'similar suffering'; to cure like with like. This is a fundamental concept in homoeopathic medicine, intrinsically borne in the very name which Samuel Hahnemann gave to the new method of medicinal cure which he discovered and formulated at the end of the eighteenth and beginning of the nineteenth centuries. From ancient time the art and science of medicine has always been a quest to alleviate and cure human suffering. The route by which the many discoveries in medicine have been made is an exciting and ever-changing story of courage, insight, progress, regress, synthesis: a vast saga of human endeavour. Thus, to understand homoeopathic medicine and its historical origins, I have chosen here to follow the route of medical discovery and enquiry from our European Renaissance to the age in which Hahnemann lived and, in this way, to trace the lineage of thinkers, experiments, discoveries and experiences that were the precursors to the formation of the essential concepts within homoeopathic medicine.

In looking closely at the life and work of the founder and discoverer of the homoeopathic principle, Samuel Hahnemann (1755–1843), a pattern emerges of ideas, influences, cultural realities and historical momentum behind his discoveries, showing a logic of historical evolution that led to the exact emergence of such a science.

It is too simple to look just at Samuel Hahnemann's work and say 'this is the work of one great man in a vacuum'. He was by no means in a vacuum. As the founder of homoeopathic medicine, he had partial antecedents in medical history although, of course, he discovered and synthesized all the basic and far-reaching tenets and laws of homoeopathic medicine. Biographies have been written of the man and his work[1] and a view of an isolated individual often emerges, without a totally clear historical context. Perhaps this mystification has led orthodox medicine to relegate homoeopathy to a misunder-stood position. It is important to look at why that has happened in a modern culture that seeks always to defend its materialistic origins the better to explain its materialistic existence and, by so doing, defend it from the potential explosion of its mythology. A need exists, nevertheless, in a great part of humanity not only to discover truths but to cure itself of its suffering.

In *The Structure of Scientific Revolutions*[2] Thomas S. Kuhn analyses facets of transformation in scientific thought and practice, albeit relating them specifically to enormous moments of change in scientific development – such as the works of Copernicus, Newton or Einstein. He shows very clearly that the history of science cannot be seen just as a linear, accumulative process. So, too, with the history of medicine. In discussing the revolutionary nature of the moments of change within scientific discovery, he points out:

> That is why a new theory, however special its range of application, is seldom or never just an increment to what is already known. Its assimilation requires the reconstruction of prior theory and the re-evaluation of prior fact, an intrinsically revolutionary process that is seldom completed by a single man, and never overnight. No wonder historians have had difficulty in dating precisely this extended process that their vocabulary impels them to view as an isolated event.[3]

The emergence of homoeopathic medicine is not unlike any other scientific reality in that it was not only revolutionary medically in its time of discovery but still represents a revolution of thought in its approach to illness. Not only did its theories, practice and methods propose a radical change from the medicine being practised in Hahnemann's lifetime but they still represent a view of reality somewhat at loggerheads with contemporary scientific and medical beliefs. Thomas Kuhn does, however, discuss the nature of crisis in the formation of all scientific revolutions. That crisis in the practice of a particular form is a prerequisite for the necessary discovery of a new method. The process is always complex, both rejecting the old and reabsorbing past notions while, simultaneously, creating a new synthesis or a totally new method. Thus we are also looking in medical science at the dialogue between the specific context of 'need' in a culture, how an individual medical man or group of practitioners respond to that need, and the knowledge available to them by which to fill that need.

There are a number of key figures in the drama of the evolution of medicine in this precise sense, from the Renaissance up to Hahnemann's day, and certainly well before. But the period from the Renaissance to the nineteenth century will be considered here rather than an overview of the whole of medical history.

Samuel Hahnemann, as well as being a medical doctor, was a linguist of some ability, a chemist of great ability, and was very involved with the history and development of medicine. He spent a great deal of the early part of his working life translating past medical texts and enquiring into the structure of the medicine he had been taught, primarily at Leipzig and Vienna. Massive dissatisfaction with the methods being used at the time led him, over years, to conduct more enquiries, research and experiments. His discovery and application of the homoeo-pathic principle and its laws emerged out of a crisis in the medical practice of his period.

As with all scientific discovery, a breakdown in the methods to achieve a given goal led a great experimenter to persist until his goal was fully attained. Hahnemann's greatest dis-satisfaction was with what he chose to call 'allopathic' medicine (from the Greek *allos* meaning 'other'), to designate

3

curing with opposites, that is, the medicine being practised by the orthodox school of medicine of his day.

At the present time, homoeopathic medicine is undergoing a new renaissance. Not only are we seeing a greater demand for this form of medicine by the public, but also a growing number of practitioners in many countries, a response again to a crisis in orthodox medicine which is not limited to medicine alone but is of a deeper and more universal nature. Homoeopathy is a corpus of medical thought and practice that has remained unscathed by the need for greater and greater dependence on technological invention. And yet, homoeopaths are fully aware of the systems of allopathic medicine and modern scientific research. Many of its critics would like to hypothesize that it is not as 'scientific' a method as allopathic medicine, inasmuch as its basic laws and tenets have not radically altered since Hahnemann's day, whilst allopathic medicine has constantly altered its frame of reference as discoveries, tools of the trade and invention of drugs change with great rapidity. Homoeopathic medicine, however, has evolved through the discoveries of its many great practitioners, building a constantly expanding homoeopathic corpus of clinical and theoretical information. It is not a static form by any means, rather an expanding one based, however, on very precise laws of cure which prove as valid today as when they were originally formulated.

In Hahnemann's *Lesser Writings*[4] we find a long extract from a letter written to 'a physician of high standing on the great necessity of regeneration in medicine'. The doctor to whom he was writing was the then celebrated Hufeland, with whom Hahnemann had had a long and intimate friendship. To quote only a few small passages from it, one can find pointers to the dissatisfaction he felt with his present-day medicine, that of the late eighteenth century, out of which he laboured to discover a new method of cure.

For eighteen years I have departed from the beaten track in medicine. It was painful for me to grope in the dark, guided by our books in the treatment of the sick, to prescribe, according to this or that (fanciful) view of the nature of diseases, substances that only owed to mere opinion their place in the *materia medica*. I had conscientious scruples about treating unknown morbid states in my suffering fellow-creatures with these unknown medicines which, being powerful substances, may, if they were not exactly suitable or not, seeing that their peculiar, special actions were not yet elucidated, easily change Life into Death, or produce new affections and chronic ailments, which are often much more difficult to remove than the original disease. . . .

But whence could I obtain aid, *certain, positive* aid, with our doctrine of the powers of medicinal substances founded merely on vague observations, often only on fanciful conjecture, and with the infinite number of arbitrary views respecting disease in which our pathological works abound?

Later, in the same passage, he concluded:

No! There is a God, a good God, who is all goodness and wisdom! and surely as this is the case must there be a way of His creation whereby diseases may be seen in the right point of view, and be cured with certainty, a way not hidden in endless abstractions and fantastic speculation.

But why was it never discovered in two or two and a half thousand years during which there have been men who called themselves physicians.[5]

Hahnemann was so disillusioned with the state of medical practice and knowledge that, soon after his marriage in 1782, he totally refrained from practising medicine, having received his degree in medicine at Erlangen in 1779, so deep was his belief that the tools he had been given would do more harm than good. He concentrated on his medical translations and seemed to wait for the day when, through his studies, questioning and experimentation, a way would emerge in which he could be satisfied that no harm would come to his patients. He had a large family and soon the illnesses which his children contracted forced him to find a way, at the very least, to help them.

By 1796 he published his first 'Essay on a New Principle for Ascertaining the Curative Power of Drugs (with a Few Glances at Those Hitherto Employed)'.[6] It is a detailed essay, outlining

5

both the various methods that had been, and were still being, used medically, and his new axioms concerning the basis of the homoeopathic principle. He describes three ways in which practical medicine had attempted to relieve disorders of the human body.

The first way, to remove or destroy the fundamental cause of the disease, was the most elevated it could follow. All the imaginings and aspirations of the best physicians in all ages were directed to this object, the most worthy of the dignity of our art. But, to use a Spagyrian expression, they did not advance beyond particulars; the great philosopher's stone, the knowledge of the fundamental cause of all diseases, they never attained. And, as regards most diseases, it will remain forever concealed from human weakness....

By the second way, the symptoms present were sought to be removed by medicine which produced an opposite condition: for example, constipation by purgatives, inflamed blood by venesection (blood letting), cold and nitre; acidity in the stomach by alkalis, pains by opium... this application of remedies is proper, to the purpose, and sufficient, as long as we do not possess the above-mentioned philosopher's stone (the knowledge of the fundamental cause of each disease, and the means of its removal) or as long as we have no rapid acting specific which would extinguish the variolous infection, for instance, at its very commencement. In this case, I would call such remedies *temporary*... then this method of treatment (to oppose disease by remedies that produce an opposite state) get the name of *palliative* and is to be reprobated. In chronic diseases it only gives relief at first; subsequently stronger doses of such remedies become necessary, which cannot remove the primary disease, and thus they do more harm the longer they are employed, for reasons to be specified thereafter.

I beseech my colleagues to abandon this method *contraria contraris*, in chronic diseases, and in such acute diseases as take on a chronic character it is a deceitful bypath in the dark forest that leads to the fatal swamp.

He then proceeds, before exposing the third method, to expound on his own new method:

It were deplorable, indeed, if only chance and empirical apropos could be considered as our guides in the discovery and application of the proper, the true remedies for chronic diseases, which certainly constitute the major portion of human ills.

In order to ascertain the actions of remedial agents for the purpose of applying them to the relief of human suffering, we should trust as little as possible to chance, but go to work as rationally and as methodically as possible. We have seen that, for this object, the aid of chemistry is still imperfect and must only be resorted to with caution; that the similarity of genera of plants in the natural system, as also the similarity of genera of one genus, give but obscure hints; that the sensible properties of drugs teach us mere generalities, and these invalidated by many exceptions; that the changes that take place in the blood from the admixture of medicines teach nothing, and that the injection of the latter into the blood vessels of animals, as also the effects on animals to which medicines have been administered, is much too rude a mode of proceeding to enable us therefore to judge the finer actions of remedies.

Nothing then remains but to test the medicines we wish to investigate on the human body itself.[7]

After explaining in more detail what he means by this, the past use of such a procedure and his intentions at that time, he states his first axiom for the homoeopathic action of remedies.

But, as the key for this is still wanting, perhaps I am so fortunate as to be able to point out the principle under the guidance of which the lacunae in medicine may be filled up and the science perfected by the gradual discovery and application, on rational principles, of a suitable specific remedy of each, more especially for each chronic disease, among the hitherto known (and many still unknown) medicines. It is contained, I may say, in the following axioms.

Every powerful medicinal substance produces in the human body a kind of peculiar disease; the more powerful the medicine, the more peculiar and marked and violent the disease.

We should imitate nature, which sometimes cures a chronic disease by another and employ in the (especially chronic) disease we wish to cure, that medicine which is able to produce another very similar artificial disease, and the former will be cured; similia similibus.[8]

He then refers to his famous discovery of this principle in action.

In my additions to Cullen's Materia Medica [which he translated in 1790 and to which he made substantial additions and notes] I have already observed that bark [Cinchona bark] given in large doses to sensitive, yet healthy individuals, produces a true attack of fever, very similar to the intermittent fever and, for this reason probably, it overpowers and then cures the latter. Now, after mature experience, I add not only probably but quite certainly.[9]

The rest of the essay goes into great detail on the specifics of many remedies about which Hahnemann was already very knowledgeable. This was only the beginning of a long journey throughout his life to refine and illuminate his new method of medical practice; experimenting first with Cinchona bark and leading to the now famous first breakthrough in discovering the law of similars.

Here we have a glimpse of the true essence of homoeopathic medicine: firstly, the principle of 'like cures like' and, secondly, the crucial premise of 'proving' each medicine homoeopathically on healthy individuals. This process is used to illuminate and specify the precise reactions each medicinal substance produces in a healthy human being on all levels, mental, emotional and physical, to then be utilized to bring about a cure of those precise ills in each individual case. Hahnemann proved many substances in this way and published his results in his *Materia Medica Pura*[10]; many more substances have been proved in great detail since his day, to build a large homoeopathic *Materia Medica*, the most critical tool of homoeopathic practice. This dynamic and profound method of cure is still the basis of homoeopathic practice today.

What must be understood, as well, is the very uniqueness of each individual and their mode of expressing maladies which, it seems, only homoeopathic medicine can encompass. The very detailed and highly exact method of matching the proving of a remedy to the presenting symptoms of a patient so as to reach, accurately, the inner workings of the individual, is used to allow both a deep and a lasting cure to take place. This practice quite clearly points to the philosopher's stone of medicine (mentioned in the extracts of Hahnemann's writings already quoted), the fundamental cause of disease and the means of the removal of that cause.

Of the intrinsic individuality of the patient, Sir John Weir wrote in a paper, given to the Royal Society of Medicine in April 1933:

Hahnemann showed that homoeopathy is absolutely inconceivable without the most precise individuation. The names of diseases should never influence the physician, who has to judge and cure diseases, not by name but by the signs and symptoms of each individual patient. That, since diseases can only express their need for relief by symptoms, the totality of symptoms observed in each individual case of disease can be the only indication to guide in the choice of the remedy. Hahnemann knew no disease, only sick persons.[11]

In an earlier paper[12] Sir John Weir also speaks of Hahnemann's laws on the curative power of drugs:

And he lays down the law 'In order to cure gently, quickly, unfailingly and permanently, select for every case of disease a medicine capable of calling forth an effective similar to that which it is intended to cure.' *Similia similibus curentur.*

Now let us take a look at the journey of medical men and ideas from the Renaissance to the period in which Hahnemann worked. In this way, some light may be shed on how such ideas and practice came into existence. Nothing evolves out of a vacuum and so we can begin to unravel what is, in fact, a very complex and exciting process of discovery and evolution.

Notes

1. Richard Haehl, *Samuel Hahnemann, His Life and Work*, (trans. M.L. Wheeler & W.H.R. Grundy, ed. J.H. Clarke & F.J. Wheeler), 2 vols, 1922; Dr T.L. Bradford, *The Life and Letters of Samuel Hahnemann*, Philadelphia, Boericke and Tafel, 1895; Rosa Waugh Hobhouse, *Life of Christian Samuel Hahnemann*, London, C.W. Daniel, 1933.
2. Thomas S. Kuhn, *The Structure of Scientific Revolutions*, University of Chicago Press; *International Encyclopedia of Unity of Science*, vol. II, no. 2, 1970.
3. ibid., p.7.
4. Samuel Hahnemann, *Lesser Writings* (trans. R.E. Dudgeon), London, W. Headland, 1851.
5. ibid., pp. 581–3.
6. Hufeland, *Journal der practischen Arzneykunde*, vol. II, part iii, 1796; also in *Lesser Writings*, pp. 295–352.
7. Hahnemann, op. cit., pp. 307–9.
8. ibid., pp. 308, 311–12.
9. ibid., p. 314.
10. Hahnemann, *Materia Medica Pura* (trans. R.E. Dudgeon), vol. I, 1811 & 1823; vol. II, 1816 & 1823; vol. III, 1817 & 1825; vol. IV, 1818 & 1825; vol. V, 1826; vol. VI, 1827 English Editions; London, Homoeopathic Publishing Co., 1880, 1936.
11. Sir John Weir, 'Samuel Hahnemann and His Influence on Medical Thought', reprinted from the proceedings of the Royal Society of Medicine, vol, XXVI, April 1933, (section of the *History of Medicine*, p. 668–78) p. 12.
12. John Weir, 'The Science and Art of Homoeopathy', vol. II, 9th Quinquennial International Homoeopathic Congress, 18–23 July 1927, pp. 167–80.

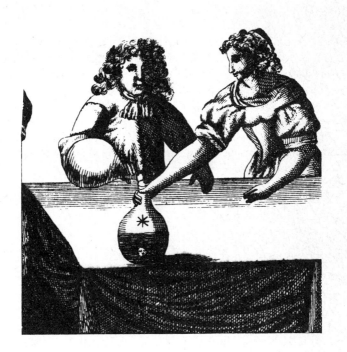

2   Paracelsus

Man is the child of two fathers – one father is the earth, the other
is heaven. . . . From the earth he receives the material body, from
heaven his character. Thus the earth moulds his shape, and then
heaven endows this shape with the light of nature. Every man
takes after his father; he is able to accomplish what is innate to
him. And the son is empowered to dispose of his paternal
inheritance.

Paracelsus

Hahnemann himself quoted Hippocrates as having written on
the law of similars. There were intimations of this idea to be
found in works of many physicians before Hahnemann.
Hahnemann, however, was the first to discover and formulate
the very exact laws of cure which gave birth to homoeopathic
medicine as a total and precise system. As is always the case with
the evolution of ideas, one cannot know and therefore examine
every minute text Hahnemann would and could have read in his
extensive study of the history and practice of medicine. What
does seem useful to analyse are the works and undoubted
influences that existed in the medical, scientific and philosophical worlds in the centuries from the European Renaissance
to Hahnemann's lifetime: the transition from early medical
alchemy, the evolution of chemistry and of early important
scientific discoveries, and the growth of greater precision, both
philosophically and scientifically, as regards man, his makeup,
his relationship to nature and to himself as an individual. There
were also times of stagnation in ideas when a cul-de-sac had
been reached in certain areas, as Hahnemann was to discover
and experience.

The evolution of ideas is always inextricably entwined with

11

the events of the world, creating them, created by them, evolving through individual crises to further plateaux of knowledge. By the time Hahnemann was studying and then practising medicine, new dissatisfactions with medical knowledge had arisen, and ideas used and experimented with in the sixteenth or seventeenth centuries no longer had the same validity.

Nevertheless, many of the discoveries made, used, rejected, transformed, would have helped to create a bedrock upon which innovation and synthesis could take place. It is often too simple to say: 'Ah . . . here is a recognizable idea two centuries before an event, this must have been an influence.' This is not always the case although, occasionally, it might be so.

Thus, I do not want to examine prior practice and theory before Hahnemann's discoveries in order to draw analogies or suppositions of this nature. Rather, I would show where seeds of thought existed, whether directly known to Hahnemann or not, to outline a pattern, a tapestry, linking various traditions and pointing to a line of thought and practice.

Various scholars and practitioners have tried to link, for instance, the work of Paracelsus (1493–1591) to that of Hahnemann. Between these two great innovators we can draw many links and conclusions and yet it is far too simple to say Hahnemann's work is a direct outcome of Paracelsus's work. That is not the case in the specific sense of Hahnemann actively paying homage to, or acknowledging, the work of Paracelsus. Richard Haehl, in his biography of Hahnemann,[1] suggests that Hahnemann refuted any connection when asked by homoeopathic followers. Nevertheless, with his extensive study of medical texts it is hard to believe he had never read the man's work or at least referred to it. And yet, although there were two and a half centuries between their lifetimes, we should look briefly at the work of Paracelsus to draw whatever conclusions seem possible.

Whether Hahnemann directly studied the work of Paracelsus or not, he would, by the turn of the eighteenth century, have reaped the results of the convoluted trajectory which the discoveries of Paracelsus had created in the medical, scientific

12

and philosophical worlds of European thought.

The contribution made by Paracelsus to the developments in medicine and science from the sixteenth century onwards was enormous. That he did not leave a totally lasting and formulated law of medical practice is also true. Without his contribution, however, his turning upside down the medicine practised in Europe of the sixteenth century, it is unlikely there would have existed a climate of ideas out of which homoeopathy and Hahnemann's work could have been produced.

While not going into great detail about the whole of Paracelsus's remarkable life and work (which I have attempted to do at a more thorough and deeper level in my forthcoming book on him, *Twelve Gates into the City*),[2] we can say that his tumultuous break with the Galenic system of medicine, practised widely throughout the Middle Ages and into the Renaissance, was of great importance in the further development of medicine.

To see more clearly exactly what Paracelsus was rebelling against, a very brief description of Galen's mode of medicine may be mentioned here.

Galen (AD 129–199) was an early Roman physician. Galenic medicine was based largely on the system of four humours, these being blood, phlegm, yellow bile and black bile, sometimes referred to as the qualities of wet, dry, hot and cold. All this was derived from Hippocrates' and Aristotle's views on the nature of man. These humours were also constitutionally known as the sanguine, the phlegmatic, the choleric and the melancholic.

To Paracelsus, Galen's system was exceptionally limited in its method of dealing with illnesses. Before examining Paracelsus's departure from that method, let us look at his major interest.

His most important interest lay in his overwhelming love and respect for nature, and experience of it. Paracelsus claimed that the physician was not a physician at all without a thorough knowledge of nature. Without any doubt, there had been physicians before Paracelsus who had observed nature, but the real axis of change, or culmination of ideas, seemed to have taken place in Paracelsus's extensive work and attitude. Above all, Paracelsus was a great naturalist, a great experimenter and a believer in medical truths being discovered through experience. Paracelsus was also a master of alchemy, having been a student of Trithemius, the Abbot of Sponheim, and a contemporary of Agrippa. He fused his alchemical knowledge with his medical practice, insisting that only those who understood the mysterious workings of nature could truly discover and make remedies useful for the medical art. Thus, in his work, we see a fusion of alchemical thought with medical practice, initiating a different view of how medicine was to be made and administered, mainly by introducing metals and minerals as important medicinal agents. Clearly, his initial understanding of chemistry was linked to the late medieval alchemists, as the application of pharmacy to medicine had been one of their contributions to the development of science. Throughout his writings one sees Paracelsus the theological and philosophical thinker. All these strains of thought led to an enormous influence on the practice of medicine, mainly after his death, and the development of the Hermetic vein of thought within certain philosophical and scientific schools. Hermetic thought embodied neo-Platonic, Judaic and Cabalistic ideas as well as magical, astrological and alchemical concepts.

Paracelsus wrote the following in *Das Zweite Buch der Grossen Wundarznei*

> The physician should be versed in all branches of philosophy, physics, and alchemy as well, as thoroughly, as profoundly as possible, and he should not lack any knowledge in these fields. What he is should stand on solid ground, founded in truthfulness and highest experience. For, of all men, the physician is supreme in the study and knowledge of nature and her light, and that is what enables him to be a helper of the sick.[3]

He believed he was undertaking the very important task of ridding medicine of the shackles and misinterpretations of the ancients, as he told his students in Basel when beginning to teach

14

there in 1527, the one brief period when he taught in an established university.

> Since medicine alone among all branches of learning is necessarily accorded the commendable title of a divine gift by the suffrage of writers both sacred and profane, and yet very few doctors deal with it felicitously at this day, it has seemed expedient to restore it to its former illustrious dignity, and to purge it as much as possible from the dross of the barbarians and from the most serious errors. We do not concern ourselves with the precepts of the ancients but with those things which we have discovered, partly by the indications found in the nature of things, and partly by our own skill, which also have been tested by use and experience. For who does not know that very many doctors at this time, to the great peril of their patients, have disgracefully failed, having blindly adhered to the dictat of Hippocrates, Galen, Avicenna and others, just as though these proceeded like oracles from the tripod of Apollo, and wherefrom they dared not diverge a finger's breadth. From these authorities, when the gods please, there may indeed be begotten persons of prodigious learning, but by no means physicians. It is not a degree, nor eloquence, nor a faculty for languages, nor the reading of many books, although these are no small adornment, that are required in a physician, but the fullest acquaintance with subjects and with mysteries, which one thing easily supplies the place of all the rest. For it is indeed the part of a rhetorician to discourse learnedly, persuade, and bring over the judge to his opinion, but it behooves the physician to know the genera, cause, and symptoms of affections, to apply his remedies unto the same with sagacity and industry, and to use all according to the best of his ability.[4]

In rebelling against the accepted dicta of Galen, which had underpinned the dominant understanding of medicine since the second century AD, Paracelsus saw serious flaws in Galenic concepts and strove throughout his life to evolve a totally new method. Galen's method had largely been based on the theories proposed earlier by Erasistratos, an Alexandrian anatomist (300 BC), coupling these with Aristotle's views on men and the Hippocratic doctrine of the four humours. The commonly held philosophical view in Galen's time, that of the Stoics, believed respiration to be the function that connected man with the cosmic spirit, that renewed his vital activities through the intake of the spiritous part of the air, the pneuma, which, in itself, was half air, half fire. But Galen believed the dominant Greek theory of his time, that all terrestrial motions were rectilinear, circular motion being only a prerogative of the celestial bodies. Thus, in his understanding of the body, there were two different kinds of blood, each with a different function, and a separate system of distribution.

Galen also placed the seats of the three vital activities of man in the digestive, respiratory and nervous systems; thus there were three functional fluids, the arterial and venous bloods, and the nervous fluid, with their controlling spirits, the vital, natural and animal. Diseases were ascribed only to internal disarrangements in the proportions of the four humours. Attempts were made, therefore, to restore the balance of the humours with medicines; these were, primarily, medicines of plant or animal origin as the humours were conceived as basically organic substances. Throughout the Middle Ages the standard practice of Galenic medicine was to administer comprehensive cure-all remedies containing as many as sixty or seventy constituents.

Galenic medicine was very much the dominant medicine practised in Paracelsus's lifetime and well into the seventeenth century. An interesting aspect of its development was the way in which, from the second century onwards, it had been taken as dogma amongst physicians in European culture and steadily became more fixed and rigid as the centuries proceeded; yet virtually no texts were available in Europe until the fourteenth century. The first printed Latin translation of substantial works of Galen was made in 1476, and the first printed Greek edition of Galen in 1525. Galenic medicine had been translated and incorporated into Arabic language and culture and formulated into their major medical practice, with occasional modifications. It was not, in fact, until the time of the height of Paracelsus's career that the definitive Aldine edition of Galen was published in Greek.

Paracelsus believed adamantly that medicine should no longer be taught solely in Latin, a language which very few understood; in this situation a tight grip on medical knowledge was held by aristocratic and university doctors. He thus insisted on teaching and writing largely in the vernacular, his own mother language being the German of Switzerland, Schweizer-Deutsch, although he wrote in High German though idiosyncratically. This was an important move on his part, to attempt to break down the rigidity and closed arena of education but, for a while, it prevented his work being widely read outside the German-speaking culture. Few of his writings were published during his lifetime, due partially to his cantankerous character and capacity to offend, and also due to the fact that some of his texts and ideas were a direct threat to established medicine and, in the case of the Fuggers (important mining owners in Austria and importers of medicinal substances from the New World), a threat to the sale of certain medicines. Paracelsus fought vigorously against the over-use of large doses of mercury in the treatment of the relatively recent scourge of syphilis. He wrote eight books on the cure of what was then called the 'French disease', but these were not to find a publisher until after his death. He posited a new way of using mercury in a milder form which was chemically altered, and specifically attacked the use of guaiac wood, imported from the New World by the Fuggers.

The full extent of the modern edition of his works comes to fourteen volumes and there are manuscripts that have not been printed. Most of his work was published some time after his death, as the interest in the Paracelsian school of thought spread and Paracelsian doctors appeared all over the continent.

Alan Debus points out in his preface to *The English Paracelsians*:

> Until recently, however, few scholars have emphasized the fact that in Paracelsus and his followers there was a curious blend of the occult and the experimental approaches to nature. These men were neither exclusively 'ancients' or 'moderns'. Rather, their work reflects strongly both ancient philosophical thought and the opening phases of the scientific revolution.

Along with their occult interpretation of the universe, the Paracelsians placed a new emphasis on chemistry as an aid to medicine, an emphasis which was to affect profoundly the development of both fields.[5]

As Paracelsus very aptly wrote:

We assume no person will doubt that the chemical art has been devised to supply the deficiencies of Nature; for, although Nature supplies very many most excellent remedies, she has, notwithstanding, produced some which are imperfect and crude; for the perfection of these a separation must be effected by which the pure is set free from the impure, so that it may at last fully manifest its powers. We desire the surgeon to be versed in this art, without which he does not indeed deserve his name. The preparation of medicaments is of great importance, so that they may be brought to their highest grade of action. God does not will that medicines should be ready too easily at hand. He has created the remedies but has ruled that they should be prepared by ourselves. The chemical art must not therefore be repudiated by the surgeon. As long as physicians are content with the preparations of the pharmacists, they will never accomplish anything worthy of praise. Furthermore, the alchemists themselves, despite the excellence of their remedies, will find their operations barren until the arts of medicine and chemistry are completely united.[6]

Paracelsus rejected the theory of the four humours as the basis of medical practice, but did not reject the concept of the four elements, fire, earth, air and water. He also introduced a new concept of the three major principles, sulphur, mercury and salt. This system of three principles had been seen in older, Islamic alchemical literature, although Paracelsus was the first to add salt as a principle. This was both a new introduction to chemical theory as well as, in Paracelsian terms, a description of spiritual substances whose properties resemble, most clearly, sulphur, mercury and salt: sulphur representing the cause of combustibility, structure and substance; salt the underlying factor behind solidity and colour; and mercury the underlying factor behind the vaporous quality. His works abound with varying versions of the relationships between the four elements and the three principles, causing some confusion during his lifetime.

To quote again from Alan Dębus:

> The value of the three principles was to be found primarily in the fact that it was a working concept. The Aristotelians talked and speculated about the four elements, but the Iatrochemists saw the vaporous, the combustible and the residuous fractions every time they ran an organic distillation.[7]

In *Philosophia de Generationibus et Fructus Quartor Elementorum*, Paracelsus wrote:

> The world is as God created it. In the beginning He made it into a body, which consists of four elements. He founded this primordial body on the trinity of mercury, sulphur and salt, and these are the three substances of which the complete body consists. For they form everything that lies in the four elements; they bear in them all the forces and faculties of perishable things.[8]

To Paracelsus, and later to the Paracelsians, the entire universe could be understood in terms of a chemical philosophy as he believed Creation itself to be a divine chemical process. Paracelsus thus saw disease as a chemical reaction within the body, different diseases arising because of the different interactions of the three fundamental principles with the four elements. He started to look at external causes for disease and to study exactly what took place in particular organs where certain diseases might be localized.

Another area where he clearly broke with Galenic tradition was to advocate the principle of like curing like. Galenic medicine always affirmed that 'contraries cure'; for instance, a medicine with an excess of the 'hot' quality would restore to balance a humoral system that was predominantly 'cold'.

Paracelsus realized that inherent in the disease process was also the nature of the cure, pointing to his understanding of the inner vitality of man as a healing force and to the similarity of the manifestation of the disease to its method of cure. We see this in his writing when he says: 'There where diseases arise, there also can one find the roots of health. For health must grow from the same root as disease, and whither health goes thither also disease must go.'[9]

In the same text he states, on curing with similars: 'Never a hot illness has been cured by something cold, nor a cold one by something hot. But it has happened that like has cured like.'[10]

In opposing the Galenic precept of treating illness with contraries, he says elsewhere:

For man is not to be understood thus, that contrary were treated with contrary, such as fire with water, but same in same. For if it were so that only something contrary would drive away a contrary, such as the fire by water, what would there then be to drive away the water? What the air? What the earth? What the winter? What the summer?[11]

Following the neo-Platonists, he argued that all that existed in man (the mircocosm) was a direct reflection of all in the universe (the macrocosm). Stemming from the Renaissance return to ancient texts, a rich school of neo-Platonic and Hermetic thought had emerged and, as a result of the fifteenth-century Florentine thinkers, was undergoing a revival in Paracelsus's lifetime. Paracelsus's deep search for the divine in nature and his persistent awareness that nature and man was a reflection of, and an emanation from, God, gave his understanding of the microcosm-macrocosm reality an intense fervour and direction.

This was clearly linked in his philosophy with his understanding of the role of alchemy. Alchemy was his tool of approach to the neo-Platonic universe. In constantly using the term 'alchemy' he imbues it with the meaning of a natural scientific method. The aspect of medieval alchemy – transmuting base metals to gold – was not his aim at all. Rather, it was to use alchemical techniques, that is, his understanding of chemistry, to discover and make efficacious remedies for medicinal use.

In *Alchemy, the Third Column of Medicine*, he states: 'It is not, as some madly assert, that Alchemy makes gold and silver. Its special work is this – to make *arcana* and direct these to disease.' *Arcana* were, to Paracelsus, the essential quality in a substance that is curative. He points out further in the same text:

> The ultimate and sole proposition is that the principle of medicine consists of these *arcana*, and that *arcana* form the basis of a physician. Now, if the sum total of the matter lies in *arcana*, it follows that the foundation of all is Alchemy, by which *arcana* are prepared. Know, therefore, that it is *arcana* alone which are strengths and virtues.[12]

With this concept Paracelsus also intermingled his understanding of planetary influences. All of nature was imbued with specific influences from specific planets and their characteristics which could similarly be reflected in the planetary influences upon exact parts of the body; thus, exact correlations could be found between a medicine and an illness. This, of course, formed part of his Hermetic view of medicine.

As he stated in the *Paragranum*:

> Medicine rests upon four pillars: philosophy, astronomy, alchemy and ethics. The first pillar is the philosophical knowledge of earth and water; the second, astronomy, supplies its full understanding of that which is of fiery and airy nature; the third is an adequate explanation of the properties of all four elements – that is to say, of the whole cosmos – and an introduction into the art of their transformation; and, finally, the fourth shows the physician those virtues which must stay with him up until his death, and it should support and complete the three other pillars.[13]

This definition of the four pillars of medicine was the basis upon which Paracelsus built his system of medicine. Within this was a precise definition for Paracelsus: that all matter proceeded from Prime Matter, which was, basically, uncreated, 'prepared by the Great Artificer Himself', which Paracelsus called

Mysterium Magnum, the generating substance from which all mysteries proceed.

He also posited within his understanding of medicine that there were specific *archei* within the body of man, ruling the physiology of the body. They related to each specific organ, the major *archeus* being that of the stomach, the alchemist of the body. Thus, disease could emanate from the improper action of the *archei*, preventing poisons from being eliminated from the body and thus resulting in disease.

Beneath all this lay his firm belief in experience being the physician's greatest tool; his love of nature, of man, and of God were also fundamental to him. On the question of the truly compassionate physician, he says: 'The art of medicine is rooted in the heart. If your heart is false, you will be a false physician; if your heart is just, you will also be a true physician.'[14]

Experience came forth through the acknowledgement and understanding of *scientia*, the essential working of all things. Knowledge was the outcome of combining *scientia* with *experientia*.

> Knowledge is *experientia* (*Erfahrung*), something we know for certain, in contrast with 'experiment', which by itself is merely accidental. The latter may be integrated with theory before it can become knowledge, the mother of experience....[15]

> Therefore, *scientia* is what is in full accord with knowledge through the just order of nature and *scientia* is contained in the object in which God provided it. *Experientia* is knowledge of cases in which *scientia* has been put to the test.[16]

It is possible to say here that we can see the early kernel of a concept of natural scientific exploration. Paracelsus's keen, almost obsessive, desire to discover the innate and beneficial secrets of nature bore definite fruit in this direction.

His experience as a physician and naturalist was varied, due to his itinerant and rebellious existence. He grew up in very close contact with nature in Eisendeln, a high mountain village in German Switzerland, under the guidance of his father, also a

22

physician. Then, at an early age, he was moved by his father whose work took him to the Fugger mines in Austria. His early fascination with, and curiosity about, nature grew and grew. Later, between 1517 and 1524, he travelled with various armies as their physician, in Holland, Scandinavia, Prussia, Tartary, countries under Venetian influence, and possibly the Near East. In this way, he gained experience of the types of illnesses and wounds inflicted by war and commonly found amongst travelling armies. At a later point still, he again returned to the Fugger mines and worked specifically with the miners and their diseases.

A major contribution by Paracelsus through his writing, learning and teaching were his new ideas on how to introduce metals and minerals into medicinal use. Until this point they had largely been considered of little value in medicine. Only the animal and vegetable kingdoms had been the source of medicinal substances. After his death one major attribute which was to distinguish his followers (often called iatrochemists) was their use of metallic and mineral medicines. The tradition of separating the pure from the impure in metals and minerals had been a concern of the medieval alchemists, but one may be able to point to the introduction of antimony, mercury and iron salts as the result of Paracelsus's authentic texts.[17] Many scholars have debated exactly when and where this precise introduction to the pharmacopoeia took place; however, enough research does seem to have been done to point to Paracelsus as a key figure in this process.

A great deal of Paracelsus's work with metals and minerals stemmed from his work and experience with mines and miners. He evolved specific theories of the way in which miners contracted diseases as a result of contact with the substances they mined. He studied the diseases the miners manifested in great detail and concluded, with very specific reference to the symptoms they produced, that the source of these illnesses was clearly a result of the exact metal contacted, both directly with the ore and via what Paracelsus called the 'fumes' from these metals. He proposed that these diseases be treated with remedies made from the exact metals which had caused the specific illnesses. In other words, he saw in these studies yet another aspect of like curing like.

What is just as important to understand in this context of Paracelsus's medical practice and philosophy is the emphasis he put on making metallic and mineral remedies via very precise methods of separation in the chemical process. We find constant reference to the use of 'quintessences' and *arcana* in his medical texts, as well as to the very exact method of making these medicines and to their use for specific illnesses. Although from our present-day understanding of chemistry and the action of medicines these recipes may seem not very fully developed, they nevertheless had a reverberating, challenging and catalytic effect on medical thinking after Paracelsus's lifetime. In later chapters we will be looking at the form these different developments took.

He also was very aware of two factors which he insisted on in the administration of medicines: the one being his concern to separate the poisonous aspect of a substance from the non-poisonous and, within that, his acknowledgement that poisons may be of medicinal use and interest; secondly, his insistence on understanding correct dosage which he knew had to be far smaller than the dosage commonly used in his time, as well as far more precisely related to the specific level of illness of the patient.

In the *Labrinthus Medicorum Errantium vom Irrgang der Arzte* he wrote:

> Is not a mystery of nature concealed even in poison? . . . What has God created that He did not bless with some great gift for the benefit of man? Why then should poison be neglected and despised, if we consider not the poison but the curative virtue? . . . And who has composed the prescriptions of nature? What is not God? . . . In His hand there abides all wisdom, and He alone knows what He puts into each *mysterium*. Why then should I be surprised and why should I let myself be frightened? Should I, because one part of a remedy contains poison, also include the other part in my contempt? Each thing should be used for its proper purpose, and we should use it without fear, for God Himself is the true physician and the true medicine. . . .

He who despises poison does not know what is hidden in i[
the *arcanum* that is contained in the poison is so blessed th[
poison can neither detract from it nor harm it.[18]

And in the same text:

In all things there is poison, and there is nothing without a
poison. It depends only upon the dose whether the poison is
poison or not... I separate that which does not belong to the
arcanum from that which is effective as the *arcanum*, and I
prescribe it in the right dose... then the recipe is correctly
made.... That which redounds to the benefit of man is not
poison; only that which is not of service to him but which injures
him is poison.[19]

Concerning the administration of remedies, Paracelsus made
yet another attack on his contemporaries whom he felt had no
accurate understanding of this process. Throughout his works
he attacked the ointment and pill makers, apothecaries and
physicians who not only used medicines that, to his mind, had
no curative effect whatsoever, but made up vast compounds of
far too many remedies with little reference to the patient or
illness being treated. In this passage Paracelsus uses his
exuberant language and alchemical symbolism to explain
correct dosage:

Remedies should not be administered according to their weight,
but according to other measurements. Who can weigh the
brilliance of the sun; who can weigh air, or the *spiritum
arcanum*? ... No one.... The remedy should operate in the
body like a fire... and its effect on the disease should be as
violent as that of fire on a pile of wood. This mystery of fire
should also apply to what you call dosage. How would it be
possible to weigh the amount of fire needed to consume a pile of
wood or a house? No, this cannot be weighed! However, you
know that one little spark is heavy enough to set a forest on fire,
a little spark that has no weight at all.... Just as the spark acts
on the wood and becomes great or small according to the
amount of it, so you must act when dealing with remedies. You
must administer them to the patient in accordance with the

extent of the illness. But who would indicate a definite weight for this? No one![20]

Paracelsus's medical writings are filled with his new principles and divisions useful for diagnosis, his understanding of the many levels at work in the patient and in disease, and long treatises on the making and administration of medicines, as well as on philosophy and theology. One vital aspect of his thinking can be seen in his description of what he called the *ens*, or active principles governing human beings. To Paracelsus, the inner man was by no means divided as such from the physical man and his ills. He saw man as a totality and yet he divided the sources of illness in different areas. He says of this:

> There are two realms into which disease can penetrate and spread. The first is that of matter, that is to say the body; it is here that all diseases lurk and dwell ... the other realm is not material; it is the spirit of the body which lives in it intangible and invisible, and which can suffer from exactly the same diseases as the body. But, because the body has no share in this life, it is the *ens spirituale*, the spiritual active principle, from which the disease springs ... therefore there are two kinds of disease: the spiritual and the material.[21]

He then divided the *ens* and defined the five divisions elsewhere in the same text:

> The *Entia*, the active principles or influences, which govern our bodies and do violence to them are the following: The stars have a force and efficacy that has power over our body so that it must always be ready to serve them. The virtue of the stars is called *ens astrorum*, and it is the first *ens* to which we are subjected. The second power that governs us and that inflicts disease upon us is *ens veneni*, the influence of poison. Even if the stars are sound and have done no injury to the subtle body in us, this *ens* can destroy us; therein we are subject to it and cannot defend ourselves against it. The third *ens* is a power that injures and weakens our body even when the two other influences are beneficient; it is the *ens naturale*, the natural constitution. If it goes astray or disintegrates, our body becomes sick. From this,

26

many other diseases can arise, even if the other *entia* are sound. The fourth *ens*, the *ens spirituale*, the spiritual entity, can destroy our bodies and bring various diseases upon us. And, even if all our *entia* are propitious to us and are sound, yet the fifth *ens*, the *ens Dei*, can make our bodies sick. Therefore none of the *entia* deserves as much attention as this last one, for by it one can recognize the nature of all other diseases . . . note moreover that the various diseases do not come from one cause but from five.

The entire works, life, philosophy and medical premises of Paracelsus are, as one can see, very complex and enormously challenging within the context of Renaissance Europe, and even to this day. He attempted to redress the balance of medicine away from that which he considered useless and profane and towards a medical system based upon a deep commitment to cure the suffering of his fellow men. His observation of nature, and the many discoveries he made during this process, were to herald an awakening of a more general scientific approach in his insistence that nature must be observed very accurately and her secrets employed to produce medicines of greater and greater efficacy. Permeating this was his philosophy based on experience – the paramount value and supremacy of experience – and his Hermetic understanding of the divine in nature and man; accompanying this philosophy was the firm belief in the theory of the macrocosm and microcosm.

In speaking of the correct 'composition' of remedies in *The Archidoxies* he says:

Concerning which Hermes Trismegistus said that it was necessary for him who intends to make this composition to create a new world; and, as God created the heaven and the earth, so also the physician must form, separate and prepare a medicinal world. And, in order that he might point out to his disciples with sufficient fidelity from what thing or material this composition should be made, and how also the concordances of heavenly virtues are discovered by us in the Valley of the Shadows, he wisely and truly adds, a little after, that what is beneath is as that which is above and that the inferior and the superior stand related to one another as man and wife.[22]

Paracelsus cannot really be separated from the age in which he lived: the Renaissance and the early Reformation. As a rebellious and determined individual, he straddled several different worlds – culling all he felt worthy from the past and making breakthroughs to the future. Often called the Luther of medicine for his reforming relationship to established medicine, one is reminded of his burning of the books of Avicenna and Galen on the night of St John's Feast in Basel in 1527, when he briefly taught there, cleansing the slate for the new medicine he wished to teach.

He supported in his own way the peasant revolts of southern Germany and was friends with Zwingli (an ardent theological reformer). In his extensive wanderings throughout Europe and the Middle East he never overlooked the sources of learning in folk medicine and the lore of gypsies and travellers. Despite his divergent views from those of the Catholic Church he, nevertheless, did not ever break with it but always had a deep love of the Mother Church. And yet, his specific understanding of Christianity was filled with mystical beliefs and his comprehension of the intrinsic autonomy of man. He was clearly not a believer in hierarchical external structures but, rather, was an iconoclast for the greater freedom of man. He expressed this belief in the following manner:

Just as the firmament with all its constellations forms a whole in itself, likewise man in himself is a free and mighty firmament; and just as the firmament rests in itself and is not ruled by any creature, the firmament of man is not ruled by other creatures but stands for itself and is free of all bonds . . . thoughts are free and are subject to no rule: on them rests the freedom of man . . . everything we invent has its origin in the spirit. Therefore, let us not concern ourselves with how things have come to us, but trust that everything is done at God's command.[23]

Paracelsus, the profoundly religious man, was always, at the basis of his quest and yearning for truth, a visionary to the last, struggling with many inner conflicts and at odds with the society in which he lived. He left a legacy of enormous stimulation and questioning to physicians, philosophers and scientists.

Even for those physicians who totally rejected, or were sceptical of, Paracelsus's new ideas and methods, what remained for them were the accounts of his amazing cures. Although many found what he wrote or said impossible to understand, or difficult to accept, they could not deny that something in his system worked. With the spread of Paracelsian medicine and Paracelsian thinking after his lifetime these new ideas were put to the test; they evolved and were incorporated in various different directions. To us now, the Paracelsian corpus is mysterious and complex and one cannot but pay homage to the courage and fiery dynamism of such a catalytic innovator.

The evident precursors of homoeopathic ideas in the work of Paracelsus are many. It was largely due to Paracelsus's involvement with a neo-Platonic, mystical-alchemical universe of the late Renaissance (he being a true 'adept') that led to his discoveries and world view. Hahnemann, however, within the context of late eighteenth and early nineteenth-century European and, specifically, Germanic culture, experienced the fruits of that mode of thinking as it had transformed through the centuries many philosophical and scientific models. Without doubt, Hahnemann lived in, and reflected, a very different period indeed.

What is so clear, however, in terms of medical ideas, was that the power for cure of the law of similars began to be realized, as did Paracelsus's insistence on small, single remedies correctly prescribed and fashioned into correct dosage. This understanding of dosage was a result of his awareness and observation of the nature of the healing force within man; he also understood that a physician must always match the exact dosage to a particular individual's malaise. His introduction of minerals and metals into the pharmacopoeia had extensive results. This will be further discussed in a later chapter on Hahnemann's discoveries and the rôle the minerals and metals play with Homoeopathic medicine.

Lastly, we cannot forget the enormous influence Paracelsus's work was to have on later generations, not just on medicine in general or on Hahnemann and homoeopathy in particular, but also on keeping alive in the medical approach the vital relationship between mind, spirit and matter; being that is the means by which disease is created and maintains itself. This influence had far-reaching, long-term effects, culminating in the work, in our century, of Carl Gustav Jung. In homoeopathy, also, we will see how important is this total relationship for understanding the individual, understanding disease, its causation and diagnosis and how to prescribe for that individual. Paracelsus's work abounds in description and observation of the psyche. He saw man as a totality and had keen observational powers (again within the alchemical framework with which he viewed reality) of the workings of the mind, spirit and emotions as they related to man's disease state and its cure.

Suffice it, therefore, to point to these discoveries, knowing that the philosophical and cultural realities of Paracelsus and Hahnemann were more than two centuries apart. There are many parallels in the work of the two men; however, to each man's discovery there exists a very specific logic, and it was clearly left to Hahnemann to perform the synthesizing of a true system of medicine, so total in its application and laws.

Which leads us to look very closely at the ways in which medicine evolved in the intervening centuries.

Notes

1. Richard Haehl, *Samuel Hahnemann, His Life and Work*, (trans. M.L. Wheeler & W.H.R. Grundy, ed. J.H. Clarke & F.J. Wheeler), 2 vols. 1922.
2. Elizabeth Danciger, *Twelve Gates into the City* (work in progress).
3. Paracelsus, *Samtliche Werke* Sudhoff Matheissen Edition, vol. 10, part I, pp. 277–8.
4. Paracelsus, *The Hermetic and Alchemical Writings of Paracelsus* (ed. Arthur Waite), London, 1894, vol. II, pp. 169–70. (Shambhala, Berkeley, 1976)
5. Alan Debus, *The English Paracelsians*, London, Oldbourne History of Science Library, 1965. ibid., pp. 9–10.
6. Paracelsus, *Chirugia Magna* (trans. Arthur Waite), tract II, ch. 9. Vol. II: *Hermetic and Alchemical Writings of Paracelsus*.
7. Debus, op. cit. p. 29.
8. Paracelsus, *Astronomia Magna*, Samtliche Werke, pp. 13,12F.
9. *Entwurte zu den vier Büchern des Opus Paramirum*, Sudhoff Matheissen Edition, p. 226.
10. *Tractatus II*, Sudhoff Matheissen Edition, I/IX, p. 236.
11. *Von Oeffnung der Haut, ein Fragment*, Liber Primus, Caput VII, Sudhoff Matheissen Edition, I/X, pp. 553–4.
12. *Alchemy, the Third Column of Medicine* (trans. Arthur Waite), vol. II, pp. 151–3.
13. *Paragranum*, Sudhoff Matheissen Edition, pp. 55–6.
14. *Von den Hinfallenden Seichtagen (de Caducis, Epilepsi) vier Paragraphen*, Erst Ansarbeitung, Sudhoff Matheissen Edition, p. 266.
15/16. Walter Pagel, *Philosophical Medicine in the Era of the Renaissance*, Basel and New York, S. Karger, 1958, pp. 59–60.
17. Debus, op. cit., p. 33.
18. Paracelsus, *Labyrinthus Medicorum*, Huser Edition, vol. I, pp. 272–4.
19. ibid., Sudhoff Matheissen Edition, pp. 136–7.
20. ibid., pp. 300–301.
21. *Das Buch von der Gebarung der empfindlichen Dinge in der*

31

Vernunft, (Von Gebarung des Menschen, Von des Menschen Eigenschaften), pp. 174–4.

22. *The Archidoxies*, (trans. Arthur Waite), pp. 90–91. (Shambhala, Berkeley, 1976).

23. S.F. Mason, *A History of the Sciences from Alchemy to Medical Chemistry*, London, Collier Books, Macmillan, 1956, pp. 232–3.

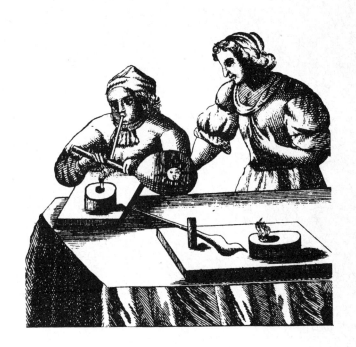

3 The Iatrochemists and the Scientific Revolution

The Paracelsians and notably Van Helmont demolished the ancient tradition throughout their whole work: It was systematically based on sound observation and experiment as well as religious and philosophical grounds: ... It is this more than anything else that reflects the watershed between the old and the new. It epitomizes the transition to a new naturalist philosophy and medicine.

Walter Pagel, *The Smiling Spleen*

Both the theories and practice of Paracelsus were of great influence during the sixteenth and seventeenth centuries, at times rivalling those of Galen. Many universities forbade the teaching of Paracelsus's works; yet, they were so popular amongst the students that, in the late sixteenth century, there were student riots in Paris and Heidelberg in protest against the prohibition of Paracelsian doctrines. With the increasing spread of his ideas, however, many physicians were willing to use 'chemically' prepared medicines, but not to incorporate Paracelsus's theories and cosmology into their work; other physicians, on the contrary, adopted his theories but not the practice, that is, the use of chemically prepared medicines.

'In his own day Paracelsus did not loom as a major figure but, after his death, a rapidly growing interest in his writings made the debate over his work one of the crucial scientific and medical problems of the late sixteenth and seventeenth centuries' comments Alan Debus.[1]

As has also been pointed out by Walter Pagel:

Enjoying a new vogue in the neo-Platonic trends of the

Renaissance, religious anti-rationalism became basic to the 'hunt for knowledge' sought by the Paracelsists. Executors to the master's heritage, they produced observations and ideas of significance in the development of modern science and medicine. At the same time they had to bear the brunt of a crisis that was played out in the seventeenth century – the debate, that is, in which leading savants and a throng of camp followers engaged in attacking, reinterpreting and redeeming the Paracelsian legacy.[2]

From the 1570s onwards a landslide of Paracelsica was reprinted, brought from the obscurity of manuscript to the wide circulation afforded by the mass medium of printing. By 1618, many Paracelsian mineral medicines were received into the London *Pharmacopoeia* in the wake of a strong international Paracelsian movement. In France, a struggle between the Paracelsians and the Galenists was quite dramatic whereas, in England, semi-official approval had been given to 'chemical' medicines by their inclusion in the *Pharmacopoeia*.

There was a prevalent dislike of a mystical approach to science amongst Englishmen at that time, and thus the occult aspects of Paracelsian thought were rejected while the new remedies were eagerly adopted, provided they proved useful in practice. It is interesting that, in the first half of the seventeenth century, there was no real English school of Paracelsianism as such. Rather, there were individuals who adopted these views. Much interest was generated by the importation and translation of Joseph Duchesne's Paracelsian work from France. Robert Fludd's work, although it showed definite understanding, and incorporation, of Paracelsian ideas, attracted very little attention in England but became well known on the continent. Thus a compromise position was upheld by many physicians in England at the end of the sixteenth and early seventeenth centuries; basically, Galenist ideas prevailed and mineral remedies were included when necessary.

As James Primerose stated (in 1638):

... though the Galenists do justly refuse the doctrine of Paracelsus, yet they do not disallow of chymicall remedies, but leave them their own place in Physick. And the Chymists themselves cannot be without remedies prepared after the vulgar way, as is evident in Quercetanus, and others, yea and Paracelsus himself, who prescribes many decoctions and infusions, and uses many things whole, not changed at all by any chemicall art. Therefore, to both of them their own praise is due; for sometimes there is need of using chymical remedies, sometimes, yea very often, the other.[3]

In France, however, a division existed between the two great schools of medicine, the one in Paris and the other in Montpellier. The Galenist faculty in Paris had the right to limit practitioners in the city to Paris graduates. The school in Montpellier, on the other hand, was becoming more and more oriented towards the iatrochemists ('iatro' in Greek meaning physician). Slowly, but surely, medical graduates from Montpellier were moving to Paris where they used metallic and mineral remedies in their practices. This annoyed the Paris faculty enormously.

The two most vociferous French iatrochemists were Joseph Duchesne and Theodore Turquet de Mayerne. Duchesne's work had a great impact on Elizabethan and Jacobean physicians. His major works, of a clear Paracelsian nature (although never mentioning Paracelsus by name), were all translated into English in the early seventeenth century by Thomas Tymme. Duchesne had studied medicine at Basel, taking his medical degree in 1573, and then moved to Paris when appointed physician to Henry IV in 1593. Ten years later he published *De Materia Verae Medicinae Philosophorum Priscorum* in which he upheld the three Paracelsian principles and opposed the Galenist doctrines and remedies. Like Paracelsus, Duchesne upheld the principle of like curing like, rather than the method of curing with contraries. He was heavily condemned almost immediately by the faculty in Paris, but he found a staunch ally and colleague in Theodore Turquet de Mayerne.

Mayerne had studied at Heidelberg and then Montpellier where he took his MD in 1597. He, too, became a physician to the King in Paris shortly after obtaining his degree. The faculty in Paris turned against him but Henry IV ignored their protests and continued to honour him. After successfully treating an influential Englishman in Paris he was invited to England where he was appointed a physician to the Queen. Mayerne, however, returned to France where he remained until the assassination of Henry IV in 1610. James I then summoned him to England and he was appointed Chief Physician to the King and his household; he retained this post until his death in 1655. During those years in England he had been influential in the compiling of the *Pharmacopoeia*. Thus it was that leading Paracelsian doctors rose to high positions and had some degree of influence.

Since the time of Paracelsus's turbulent attack on the Galenic system, other discoveries had been made, nearly as vociferous in their assault on Galenic assumptions as Paracelsus's had been, although from a very different angle. The work of Vesalius the anatomist (1514–64), Professor of Anatomy and Surgery at Padua University, was notable. He started off his energetic career as a defender of Galen and yet, the more he was able to dissect human bodies (and very difficult indeed it was to get bodies to dissect) the more he realized how erroneous Galen had been in basing his understanding of human anatomy on that of animals. Vesalius discovered that Galen believed human anatomy to be the same as that of the ape.

On every level many discoveries and changes of attitude were being made at that time. The Renaissance, the Reformation and, subsequently, the Counter-reformation had overturned the entire map of European thought and religious belief. Medicine, also, went through many enormous changes in relation to this social, religious and philosophical enquiry. Copernicus (1473–1543), who lived at the same time as Paracelsus, had truly turned the entire world upside down with his new and more accurate model of the universe, a sun-centred universe rather than an earth-centred one. Later, Galileo and Kepler were to make their important discoveries. In the midst of all this, the need in medicine to turn to experience and observation of nature was an inevitable and crucial step in the evolution of medical scientific thought. By the end of the sixteenth and beginning of the seventeenth centuries two streams of thought were emerging to challenge the accepted Galenic medical view. One set of ideas was directed towards early chemistry and influenced by

Paracelsus; the other was more mechanical in its outlook and methods. The iatrochemists or vitalists considered inorganic substances to be alive, while the mechanical philosophers considered matter to be dead and inert, undergoing change only when subject to external mechanical forces.

After Vesalius's discoveries and publication of his *Concerning the Fabric of the Human Body* in 1543, other medical men were to follow up the search for more accurate understanding of the anatomical functioning of the human body. Not until the early seventeenth century, however, did William Harvey (1578–1657), discover the true nature of the circulation of the blood. Earlier attempts by Michael Servetus (1511–53), burnt at the stake along with his books by Calvin as a heretic, and Realdo Columbo (1510–59), successor to Vesalius at Padua, had produced ideas on the lesser circulation of the blood, regarding respiration as the process which purified and vitalized the blood (rather than Galen's conception that the blood passed through the septum of the heart). But it was not until Harvey did his intensive empirical research and published his book *On the Motion of the Heart and the Blood* in 1628 that the theory of the circulation of the blood was established. Harvey's ideas broke totally with the Galenic and Aristotelian view that only celestial bodies had circular movement, while terrestrial movements had beginnings and endings. His understanding coincided with the new world view of a sun-centred universe, equating the heart with the sun and giving it primacy of importance, whereas Galen had held it to be only one of three important seats in the body, along with the brain and liver. In his book Harvey wrote:

> The heart is the beginning of Life; the sun of the microcosm, even as the sun in his turn might well be designated the heart of the world, for it is the heart by whose virtue and pulse the blood is moved, perfected, made apt to nourish, and is preserved from corruption and coagulation; it is the household divinity which, discharging its function, nourishes, cherishes, quickens the whole body and is indeed the foundation of Life, the source of all action. . . . The heart, like the prince in a kingdom, in whose hands lie the chief and highest authority, rules over all; it is the

original and foundation from which all power is derived, on which all power depends in the body.[4]

However, Harvey made it very clear that he had not based his discoveries on philosophical premises but, rather, on empirical findings. He established that the movement of the blood was circular, but he could not find the small capillaries to make it a full circle, as he did not have a microscope. In the end, he based his theory on his faith that Nature had not failed to complete the circle.

Even though these advances were crucial for the development of a modern understanding of the human body and its physiology, certain major figures in the iatrochemical school were unaware of these discoveries of Harvey's. Their researches, writings and work took them in other directions, also of importance for the development of medicine and Paracelsian ideas.

One such important figure was the Flemish nobleman, Jan Baptista Van Helmont (1578–1644). He has often been referred to as the man whose work formed the basis of the iatrochemical school of the seventeenth century. His re-statement and re-working of the chemical philosophy was of great influence at that time. Violently anti-Galenist, like Paracelsus, influenced by him and very much in his mould, he also sought to overthrow the existing method of medical teaching and replace it with a vitalistic philosophy based on theological and natural truths. His emphasis was always on experimental and observational data. It could be said that he was one of the most important chemical philosophers of the seventeenth century.

He received his medical degree at Louvain in 1599 and then travelled for several years, albeit being offered posts in various courts. But, after his marriage in 1609, he decided to retreat in order to study. He wrote in *Promissa Autoris*:

I withdrew myself from the common people to Vilourd that, being less troubled, I might proceed diligently to view the kingdom of vegetables, animals and minerals by a curious Analysis, or unfolding, by opening bodies and separating all things. I went about my search for full seven years. I searched into the books of Paracelsus, filled in all parts with a mocking obscurity or difficulty, and I admired that man and too much honoured him till at length understanding was given of his works and errors.[5]

Van Helmont completely rejected the Galenist theory of humours and, with it, also rejected the use of contraries in medical practice as he saw the one to be an extension of the other. He believed that the predominance of doctrines based on 'polarity' and 'contraries' prevented the development of real science and truth and had a particularly destructive influence on medicine. He was not, however, fully in accord with Paracelsus's understanding of the use of similars, nor was he totally convinced of the three principles – salt, mercury and sulphur – that had been put forward by Paracelsus. He believed water to be the most important and basic element, the primary matter, and he did extensive experiments to try to prove this. He felt the function of the elements and principles had been misunderstood. While also not accepting the full theory of microcosm-macrocosm as understood by Paracelsus, specifically in the area of the influence of the stars on man's health, he did, however, see the 'divine chemical' understanding of nature as crucial. His approach to nature was indecipherable without a knowledge of chemistry. It is in this area and in the use of the concept of the *archeus*, within his basically vitalistic and religious approach, that we see him as similar to Paracelsus; indeed, his work directly evolved from that of Paracelsus into a more refined and practical synthesis.

To Paracelsus, the *archeus* was an essential concept in his understanding of the human being. It was the innate vital force, the inner healer of the being, invisible and yet extremely important. In all places where the *Spiritus Vitae* and the immaterial principle of life could be found, the *archeus* was represented. According to Paracelsus, the *archeus* is the vital principle of *anima mundi*, that which directs and maintains the growth and continuation of living things. The *archeus* in the human body separated the useful from the useless in ingested food and transformed nutrient into body tissue, very like a miniature alchemist inside the laboratory of the human frame. There were, in his view, subsidiary *archei* of particular organs, and disease could be quelled by the *archeus* of the mineral or plant that provided the specific remedy.

Van Helmont, like Paracelsus, believed that disease could be defined as an affair of the *archeus*. Disease could be generated by the *archeus*, take place in it, and the outcome of the disease depended on it. By the *archeus*, Van Helmont meant the 'vital principle', that which governs the whole of the organism. He believed the *archeus* to have its seat in the spleen, controlling all the physiological processes of sickness and health. The *archeus* was, to him, as it had been to Paracelsus, a vital and spiritual force. It was not the 'Soul', however. 'It is the psychic aspect of a specific living unit, an individual. As such, it is inseparably interlocked with its material and bodily aspect....'[6]

Coupled with this understanding of the *archeus* was a definition of disease in a world composed of innumerable 'seeds' or *semina*, which are neither spirit nor matter, but something of both. They are at the origin of all things, and thus also of disease. These *semina* were, however, primarily spiritual and invisible.

'It is these vital *semina* with their complicated psycho-physical structure which Van Helmont wanted to set up in contrast to the traditional terms of heat and humours.'[7]

He rejected the notion of heat being a vital factor governing living structures and their functioning; he felt, rather, that heat was a companion of life, a sign of the *modus operandi* in warm-blooded animals.

These 'seeds' of disease were made active and fertile by an imaginative process by which an image of the disease was conceived. These particular acts generated by the imagination were located in the *archeus*. Van Helmont held the idea of *semina* exactly in common with Paracelsus, for they both posited that disease springs from specific 'seeds'. Van Helmont believed that there was a real and essential interaction between an outside agent and a disease image. Not that the outside agent was made of particles of foreign 'stuff', but rather that the *archeus*, the immanent spiritual force of each object, could affect another *archeus* and so cause disease.

> He believed he had made evident the *archeus* when he deprived an object of its coarse material cover 'through fire' and obtained a smoke with properties specific to the object. In this he saw its purest form, its divine kernel. He called the smoke with the 'new form' Gas, as different from such general media as air and water vapour. This is indeed the gas of our modern textbooks of chemistry, and Van Helmont is rightly remembered as its discoverer. To him, however, Gas meant much more – it was the *archeus* that vitalized all objects, notably those of organic nature.[8]

Within his concept of the *archeus* and the role an image or idea of a disease played, Van Helmont made it clear that he believed disease to proceed from spirit to matter. In his work *Oriatrike* he says, 'the *archeus* frames erroneous images to himself which should be unto him as it were for a poison... which images or likenesses, indeed, as being the seeds of disease beings, should be thenceforth wholly marriageable unto him in the innermost bride-bed of life'.[9] Later, in the same text, he says, 'And so every disease is caused from the violent assaulting spirit, by ideas conceived in the proper subject of the *archeus*, by whose fault alone a live body, but not a dead carcass, suffers all diseases.'[10]

With the spirit of empiricism and reliance on experience embedded in his work and outlook, Van Helmont pointed out: 'We do not know other natures *a priori*, but only by naked observation, and the alterations of the *archeus* in the same way.'[11] He called himself a 'Hippocratic and Hermetic physician' in a work published in 1624, pointing to the fact that he had immersed himself in a study of Hippocrates's work and had also been very influenced by neo-Platonic thinking. In this vein, like Paracelsus before him, he considered 'logical' thinking of little use, rather 'understanding' to be of paramount importance. On this specific point – his emphasis on understanding rather than reason and logic – Harris Coulter points out:

He realised that it emerges from a mixture of memory, reason, imagination and will which he would 'rather experience than determine'. But his great contribution was to cast this new knowledge in the Platonic form of recollection or pre-existing ideas – thus according the new scientific knowledge a privileged position in the world of discourse. In so doing, he expanded the empirical definition of knowledge as observation and experience preserved in the memory. While accepting this definition, he extrapolated from it, using it as a vehicle to justify the emergence of a new form of knowledge by fusing it with the Platonic recollection (memory) of eternal Ideas.[12]

Relying on experience as his guide and understanding as his key to illness, Van Helmont saw disease in a very specific light. 'I do not know epilepsy, lepra, apoplexy – I only know individuals, epileptics, lepers, apoplectics. For disease only exists as a modification of Life. There are no diseases, there are only sick men.'[13] He considered outside agents to be 'occasional causes' rather than the essence of disease. As a student of anatomy, physiology, and pathology, Van Helmont rejected the idea of catarrh which was generally accepted at that time to account for disease. Vapours were alleged to rise from the stomach to the brain where they condensed to a mucus that then flowed down the base of the skull to all parts of the body. The result, according to Galenist doctors, was pneumonia or consumption in the lungs; rheumatism and gout in the joints; and ulceration in the legs. This concept was closely linked to humoral pathology and it was thought that disease was caused by a surplus of corroding fluid. Van Helmont, on the contrary, did not accept this view but, rather, believed that disease was caused by specific 'seeds' which had unique and individual cycles and localized causes relating to the *archei* and their influence. No illness could develop, according to Van Helmont, where there was not a sympathetic relationship between the alien *archeus* and that of the host.

This idea of sympathetic action permeates the whole of his work.

As far as Van Helmont could see, the prevalent form of medical practice lacked precision on almost every level. In the main, he could not see any precision in the relationship of the use of remedies to specific illnesses and patients, nor an adequate knowledge of the sources of medicines. He saw his fellow practitioners duped by the Galenist theory of contraries and humoral thinking, and unconcerned about truly curing their patients. He often commented on how they were more interested in gain than in charity and love for their patients. This he coupled with their reluctance or outright refusal to learn from experience and their all too easy acceptance of the theories and dictums of the 'schools'. Van Helmont was violently opposed to bloodletting and the many other harsh methods used by the Galenists. As he pointed out, once again in the *Oriatrike*:

> For seeing that besides cutting of vein and the shop of laxatives, the Schools as yet to this day do scarce acknowledge other remedies, and all their endeavour is that blood, dung, bath, a cautery, sweat, and so not but by the diminishing of the body and its strength, and likewise the corrupting of blood (which they call a purge) and by miserable butchery they do presume to take away all griefs of the body. Hence it comes to pass that . . . the admirers of those frail effects have erected a plenteous company of incurable diseases . . . and have brought in a dissembling kind of cure, full of calamity and despair.'[14]

In this critique he also saw that Galenist physicians were not interested in the causes of illness, knowing little about them. He felt they were only treating the products of disease, not its root. In talking of bloodletting in this context he says again: 'The repetition of purges are vain and hurtful, and hurtful in their effects because they are those things which are appointed only about the products, but not the causes . . . the former causes or roots they are not able to touch.'[15]

And, later, in the same text he comments:

> He therefore labours for the most part in vain who . . . doth place his endeavour in brushing away the occasional causes, the *archeus* being not appeased . . . for it happens unto him no otherwise than as he who having not first stopped up the spring head presumes by exhausting of water to dry up the brook.[16]

As we can see, Paracelsus's thought and world view had a strong influence on Van Helmont's attitude, despite the few points with which he was in disagreement. The overwhelming desire on Van Helmont's part to rid medicine of its fruitless, often harmful and barbaric practices, was a strong force in him, as it was in Paracelsus. They both relied enormously on their belief in God and the divine intention that men should discover true methods by which to cure illness. Both had an overriding faith in Christian charity and 'Christian' behaviour towards their fellow men. Both also attracted constant criticism of their work and attitudes. Van Helmont has often been derided, as he was during his lifetime, for what was considered the 'occult' aspects of his work, to such an extent that the Inquisition called him for questioning in 1627. On this first occasion, he was questioned on two tracts he had written, the one defending the the 'weapon slave' (a Paracelsian legacy – of using blood from a wound on a sword to sympathetically heal the wound) and the second defending the virtue of spa waters. At this first confrontation with the Inquisition, he repented his errors and was allowed to go free and to continue his work. Before long, however, he was arrested again in 1634. This time all his papers and books were seized. He was charged by the Ecclesiastical Court with having departed from the 'true philosophy' to espouse superstition, magic and the diabolical art. Above all, he was accused of having followed Paracelsus and his disciples in preaching the 'chemical philosophy' and having thus spread the 'Cimmerian darkness' over the world. He was then placed under house arrest for two years.

By 1642 he obtained an ecclesiastical imprimatur to publish his third published work, *Febrium Doctrina Inaudita*. In 1644 the next text was published, *Opuscula Medica Inaudita*; this included work on fevers, the stone and the plague, as well as an attack on the deception and ignorance of physicians who subscribed to humoral pathology.

In this same year, Van Helmont contracted pleurisy and, knowing that his death was imminent, asked his son to compile all his works, whether corrected or not. He died a few days later, at the end of December 1644. His son, Franciscus Mercurius

Van Helmont (1618–99), a medical philosopher in his own right, did compile his father's full works and they were to appear in 1648 as the *Ortus Medicinae*, containing a new edition of the *Opuscula Medica Inaudita*. According to various medical historians, these two works proved to be amongst the most influential medical and scientific publications of the seventeenth century. As an example of how in demand they were, the Latin text was republished in 1651, 1665, 1667, 1682 and 1707, whilst they were translated into English in 1662 and 1664, into French in 1671, and then into German in 1683.

Van Helmont had accepted four different sources for medicine that could be used justifiably and successfully. The one was herbal and folk medicine; the second was chemical medicines; the third was the Paracelsian *arcana*; and, lastly, he sought to discover the specifics himself. The herbal remedies, or the simples, were a source of great study for Van Helmont. He mentioned at one point that a whole man's life could be dedicated to the study of these, as the extent of their powers to heal the sick had by no means been fully understood.

He wrote about such remedies as Agnus Castus, used as a diuretic; Helleborus Niger, for coughs and catarrh; Bryonia Alba, for dropsy; and Symphytum, for broken bones – all these were later fully extended in their use as homoeopathic remedies. Of the new chemical medicines, whose sources were mainly from the world of minerals and metals, he said: Alchemy has 'long since indeed observed a noble treasure of healing to lay hid in minerals, but it long doubted in what respect they might most fully derive themselves into the inward buttery of similar parts'.[17]

He held the Paracelsian *arcana* very highly, believing many of them to be capable of curing all diseases. Amongst a few which he employed were Elixir proprietatis, Mercurius vivus, tincture of Antimony, Mercurius diaphoreticus, Liquor alkahest; and volatile salts of various herbs and stones.

As for his specifics, he realized that the best way to ascertain them was to observe the very precise effects they had, and thus to come to understand their powers. By observing their effects on sick people, the physician could then learn best how to use his medicines. He did many experiments in this area to prove precise points and to clarify the exact relationship between remedies and diseases.

On this point he commented in the *Oriatrike*:

For the knowledge of diseases containeth the knowledge (*scientiam*) of the causes, the dependence and appropriating the same to our defensive faculties. . . . But the finding out (*inventio*) of the remedy doth presuppose the aforesaid knowledges (*cognitiones*) and, moreover, of the faculties and powers, I say, the manner and means of acting.[18]

He clearly saw disease as unique to each individual, only using the names of diseases in his writings for convenience's sake. He also understood each medicine as a unique whole, thus, like Paracelsus, advocating the use of only one medicine at a time. Also, like Paracelsus, he saw a great value in poisons which could make excellent medicines if suitably transformed. He also, interestingly, saw the role that fear could play in the creation of a disease:

A fear of the plague causes the plague; a sudden fear of death has oftentimes killed the gout. Likewise, the fear of honour lost, or to be lost, if it hath endured for the space of one day, hath now and then caused the falling sickness [epilepsy].[19]

Thus we can see that, by the middle of the seventeenth century, many of Paracelsus's ideas had been taken up, expanded, rejected or given great stimulus to further research and extrapolation. In the iatrochemists in general, and in Van Helmont specifically, we see a true continuation of Paracelsian ideas. As Walter Pagel has commented: 'The key figure in the course of Paracelsianism to secular reception and influence is Jan Baptista Van Helmont.'[20]

Many events had transpired on social, religious or philosophical levels from the time of Paracelsus's death to the middle of the seventeenth century. The advent of mechanistic thinking grew apace in certain areas of science alongside the developments just described. Amongst the great men of science of the seventeenth century, Bacon and Sir Isaac Newton (to name but two), the link with the alchemical tradition still persisted very strongly, despite the commonly held twentieth century view that these men , only promoted the new understandings of gravity, physics and mechanistic thinking as understood until Einstein shattered many concepts. The very close link between Nature, God and the new scientific exploration was a live and major factor in the medicine and science of the seventeenth century.

In her book, *The Rosicrucian Enlightenment*, Frances Yates points out, in an in-depth analysis of her subject,

> ... that the Hermetic-Cabalistic tradition as a force in the background of Renaissance science did not lose that force with the coming of the scientific revolution ... it was still present in the background of the minds of figures formerly taken as fully representative of complete emergence from such influences.[21]

Notes

1. Alan Debus, *The Chemical Philosophy*, vol. 2, New York, Science History Publications, 1977, ch. 1 'Paracelsian Science and Medicine in the Sixteenth and Seventeenth Century', p. 542.
2. Walter Pagel, *The Smiling Spleen. Paracelsianism under Storm and Stress*, Basel, S. Karger, 1984, p. 5.
3. Debus, *The English Paracelsians*, pp.175–6; also *Popular Errors or the Errors of the People in Physick* (trans. Robert Wittie), London, 1651, pp. 222–3. (London, Oldbourne, 1975)
4. S.F. Mason, *A History of the Sciences from Alchemy to Medical Chemistry*, London, Collier Books, Macmillan, 1956, pp. 220–21.
5. J.B. Van Helmont, *Ortus Medicinae,* 1648, p. 12; *Oriatrike, or Physick Refined*, London, 1662, p. 7.
6. Pagel, 'Van Helmont's Concept of Disease – To be or not to be? The Influence of Paracelsus', *Bulletin of the History of Medicine*, vol. XLVI, no. 5, Sept.–Oct. 1972, p. 422.
7. ibid., p. 426.
8. ibid., p. 422.
9. Van Helmont, *Oriatrike*, London, 1662, p. 535.
10. ibid., p. 534.
11. ibid., p. 459.
12. Harris Coulter, *Divided Legacy. A History of the Schism in Medical Thought*, vol. II, Washington, Wehawken Book Co., 1977, pp. 25–6.
13. Pagel, 'Van Helmont's Concept of Disease', *Bulletin of the History of Medicine*, vol. XLVI, no. 5, Sept.–Oct. 1972.
14. Van Helmont, *Oriatrike*, London, 1662, p. 3.
15. ibid., p. 431.
16. ibid., p. 554.
17. ibid., p. 580.
18. ibid., p. 4.
19. ibid., p. 652.
20. Pagel, *The Smiling Spleen,* Basel, S. Karger, 1984.
21. Frances Yates, *The Rosicrucian Enlightenment*, London, Paladin, 1975, p. 277.

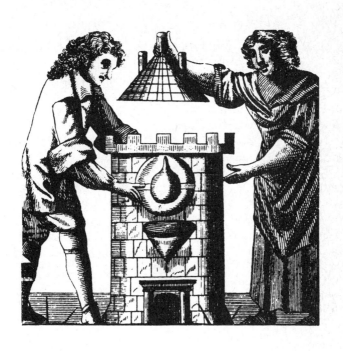

4   The Rosicrucian Element

For they (the true Alchemists), *being lovers* of Wisdom *more than*
Worldly Wealth, *drove at* higher *and more* excellent Operations.
Theatrum Chemicum Britannicum Fama Fraternitatis,
first Rosicrucian Manifesto

And certainly He to whom the whole Course *of* Nature *lyes
open, rejoyceth not so much that he can make* Gold and Silver,
or the Divells *to become* subject *to him, as that he sees the*
Heavens *open, the* Angells of God *Ascending and Descending,
and that his own Name is fairly written in the* Book of Life.

What does 'Rosicrucian' mean? It is a term much misused and,
in the twentieth century, generally employed only to describe an
esoteric group. It will be considered here as an historical
phenomenon of the early seventeenth century. In this context
will be examined the nature of the figures associated with the
Rosicrucian movement, its literature, visual emblems, allegories
and their relationship to the alchemical strain present in
medicine and science.

   In seventeenth-century Europe Rosicrucian thought crossed
geographical and language barriers, and often carried import of
both a political, spiritual and medical nature from country to
country. Its influence was felt, either through interest or
through rejection, by many of the 'great' minds of the scientific
and medical revolutions of that period.

   A noteworthy expansion of Paracelsian ideas plainly
stemmed from the same impulse although, naturally, these ideas
took slightly diverse forms. The people who carried these
thoughts were not unknown to each other though they lived in
different lands and therefore worked within different environ-

ments. As a common factor, almost all of them were Paracelsian doctors and, if not actually practising medicine, saw themselves as involved with the Paracelsian legacy.

In the introduction to her book, *The Rosicrucian Enlightenment*, Frances Yates states:

> New approaches to the history of science have revealed that the scientific advances of the Renaissance and early modern period arose in the context of a tremendous movement of religious interest in the world of nature as a manifestation of the divine, a movement in which influences which today would be labelled 'Hermetic' or 'esoteric' played a part.[1]

The Rosicrucians included, amongst their number, John Dee (1527–1608) and Robert Fludd (1574–1637), both Englishmen of great and somewhat controversial repute. In Germany there was Michael Maier (1568–1622) who was influential in Heidelberg where alchemical and Rosicrucian texts were published by De Brys and others. In this regard Francis Bacon and Sir Isaac Newton must be mentioned, though they are not directly linked to what Frances Yates called the 'Rosicrucian Furore', whereas they *were* linked to the alchemical mode of thinking.

At that time a series of links formed an almost invisible lineage of ideas connected in part to the Renaissance figure of the *magus*. Certainly, John Dee and, later, Robert Fludd were condemned on this score; the *magus* dealt with numbers and angelic or demonic forces and was, consequently, feared.

Much has been written about these men, both in the form of biography and historical analysis. Of especial value to us here is the way in which their work carried torches of change for medicine and science and, specifically, carried them forward within the spiritual and religious side of alchemy.

We cannot forget that, with the Reformation and the Thirty Years War (1618–48), the early seventeenth century was marked by the rise of Church reaction. With it came an intensified re-enactment of witch-hunts throughout Europe. That attitude led to the need, expressed by societies undergoing enormous change, to root out all that was threatening to political and social order, whatever form it took. Thus, too, the growing interest in secrecy and veiled allegory, and the symbolic forms of communication across borders via visual images or manifestos, as seen in the Rosicrucian manifestos. For 'science' to be born out of any continuous process of research into 'nature', it seems that tumult necessarily accompanies change.

As we have seen, Van Helmont was hauled up before the Inquisition of the mid-seventeenth century at the height of the Counter-reformation. He, himself, was a Catholic. Many other Rosicrucians were Protestant, Lutheran or of other denominations. Heidelberg was a seat of Lutheranism until the Counter-reformation swept it away and the city was taken in 1620 from the Elector of the Palatinate. Both hidden and overt connections with British thinkers reached European seats of learning and an interchange of ideas was continuous in the early part of the seventeenth century.

As mentioned in the previous chapter, Robert Fludd did not find a publisher for his work in England. Michael Maier, however, arranged its publication by De Brys. Fludd was much sought after, for his knowledge, in European capitals and frequently travelled there, spending long periods on the continent. John Dee, before him, had taught on the continent and had a large influence on many towards the end of the sixteenth century; he was particularly favoured by mathematicians, as that was his major concern, but he also had a following amongst philosophers, astronomers and astrologers. He avowed Pythagorean principles and developed his own language of mathematics connected, intrinsically, with his model of hierarchies of angelic forces and magical practices.

To quote from Peter French's excellent book on John Dee:

With the advent of the Reformation in England the humanist tradition became ever more drily rhetorical. The new humanism was by no means hospitable to John Dee, who was decidedly out of place in sixteenth century England. He questioned the accepted values of his time. Moreover, his Hermetic Platonism, with its magic and mysticism, seemed subversive. Dee was in the tradition stemming from Ficino, rather than in the one stemming from Petrarch. When rhetorical humanism had become highly developed in the fifteenth century, the next great discovery of the Renaissance occurred: the recovery of Greek texts with their philosophical and scientific revelations. In what might be termed the Hellenic movement, Ficino and followers like Pico della Mirandola believed they were restoring philosophy as part of a broad return to the classical world. Placing rather strict limits on the value of earlier rhetorical humanism, they emphasized philosophy, theology and science and perceived the universe in a new way with ancient wisdom as a guide. When dealing with Renaissance thought, therefore, it must be clearly recognized that humanism appealed to one type of mind, and Ficiniam neo-Platonism appealed to another type.[2]

In Dr Thomas Smith's *The Life of John Dee,* written in 1908, there is an interesting, brief description of John Dee's early life which throws some light on his background and the ambience in which he grew up.

John Dee first drew the breath of life at London on the 13th day of the month of July, at 4:00 o clock and II minutes p.m. in the year of the eternal incarnated Word 1527. His father was Roland Dee, an honourable man, and coming of a family sufficiently genteel, whose care, according to the affection implanted by nature towards his own son, as well as being a boy of great hope and good disposition, was chiefly bestowed in informing his mind with Greek and Latin literature. The curriculum of the studies in which boys are accustomed to be taught being happily passed, partly in London, partly in Chelmsford in the County of Essex, he was entered by his most loving father in his sixteenth year of his age, at Cambridge, in the college dedicated to the memory of St. John the Evangelist, to be taught the higher sciences, at the end of the year 1542.[3]

This is but a brief glimpse into the life of an Englishman of that period, his mind and attitude trained and formed by his father's intent to allow his son to pursue study and to acquire knowledge. Later, Dee was to write in the preface to *Monas Hieroglyphica* (1564), when describing the 'true philosopher' or

52

magus, saying

> Of those... who devote themselves wholeheartedly to philosophy you may hardly be able to name but one who has even had the first taste of the fundamental truths of natural science. Yet the republic of letters can muster only one man out of a thousand, even of them scholars, who have entirely dedicated themselves to study of wisdom, who has intimately and thoroughly explored the explanations of the celestial influences and events (as well as) the reasons of the rise, the condition, and the decline of other things.[4]

Dee was appointed by Queen Elizabeth I as her Astrologer Royal and Councillor on matters of state and scientific importance. His prominence and influence in Elizabethan culture was large, therefore, and yet he has been pushed aside more often than not by historians and relegated to the heap of 'magicians' to be ignored or repudiated. This may in part be due to James I's analysis of him, while Dee was still alive, as merely a magician to be tolerated and 'allowed' to live but, otherwise, to be regarded with disfavour. James I's book on demonology became a text-book for witch-hunters. It is only in this century that any serious look at Dee's work and contribution has been made.

In the late sixteenth century John Dee had an enormous influence on scientific, medical and alchemical thought, as well as that pertaining to astronomy, geography or philosophy. He was a Renaissance scholar, of equal importance to many of the great minds of his period. From contemporary accounts he was an impressive teacher. His talents were admired and supported by royalty and nobility. This is an interesting fact, in as much as the influence of royalty and the nobility in many European countries was still supreme. Thus, as was the case for so many English hermetic thinkers of that time, European capitals were a refuge for learning and teaching. In England, however, the new humanistic and mechanical philosophy moved more and more into favour.

There were several routes of learning in Europe. These encompassed the cities of London, Heidelberg, Paris and Prague and a few other offshoots, such as Strasburg. Knowledge was effected through publishers, patrons and changes arising from the Reformation and the Catholic counter-reaction.

What, then, was the Rosicrucian link?

A major link was John Dee. The actual Rosicrucian texts and manifestos were not published until the early seventeenth century in Heidelberg after John Dee's death in 1608. What is important about Dee was his prime influence on Rosicrucian thinking in that he kept the Hermetic tradition alive and thus enabled it to be applied to burgeoning scientific discourses, medical discoveries and changes in method and attitude in astronomy, physics, geography and pure philosophy. This tradition emanated from the new neo-Platonism of Ficino and the Florentine school. Within Elizabethan England in the late sixteenth century, and Europe in the early seventeenth century, the tradition became partially eclipsed but it was still a definite force in intellectual circles.

We, in the twentieth century, do not clearly see the connection to this tradition, but it is there. It is almost impossible to divide development of thought into opposing camps, although martyrs may have existed in the one and the more rigid mechanistic thinkers in the other. Discovery in any field often moves between opposites, to then find its new formulation. The late sixteenth and early seventeenth centuries were far too dramatic, creative and changeable to trace divisions too rigidly, although they surely existed. An antagonism to the Hermetic vein of thought was clearly on the increase and had an aspect of rigidifying institutional thought so as to better control diverse and enquiring ideas which led to many of the witch-hunts and burnings. Wars, pestilence, disease, dissent, changing religions and social values, alteration of the very institutions of religion and education, gave rise to an upsurge of a need to cast some rational light on important matters, especially education, science and health.

The remarkable Rosicrucian imprint was largely an impulse of this kind with very high ideals; it was a desire for all men to learn and for all men to have access to the experience of the divine in nature and the reality of a relationship with the

Godhead. The author of the manifestoes have never been fully determined; veiled secrecy accompanied the entire effort which took place over a short span of years (1614–21).

The symbolism of the Rosy Cross and the symbolism of the 'pure' individual seeking truth and wisdom was an identifiable clement in all Rosicrucian texts. There are clear elements in the manifestos of a revival of knowledge in a very accurate form; a desire to regenerate learning, discovery and communication. Francis Bacon and Sir Isaac Newton certainly followed in these footsteps with their very deep belief that learning was of fundamental importance to a good society. There was a constant search by scholars to find or contact these Rosicrucian Brothers but, as far as we know, no one was ever able to find them, according to available written sources.

A sequence of very precise Rosicrucian manifestos put forward these new ideas, couched in allegorical terms and referring to Christian mythology and theology. The Christian Rosencreutz legend and his discoveries of hidden knowledge lit by an inner light of an inner sun is central to the theme of all the documents. Paracelsus figures as an idealized personage in these texts, connected to the discovery of ancient wisdom, a precursor of the new philosophy and an inspirational force behind the drive to consolidate the continuance of this search for a regeneration of ideas. In her book, *The Rosicrucian Enlightenment*, Frances Yates comments on the first of the manifestos, the *Fama Fraternitatis*.

This very peculiar document, the *Fama Fraternitatis*, thus seems to recount, through the allegory of the vault, the discovery of the new, or rather new-old philosophy, primarily alchemical and related to medicine and healing, but also concerned with number and geometry and with the production of mechanical marvels. It represents, not only an advancement of learning, but above all an illumination of a religious and spiritual nature. This new philosophy is about to be revealed to the world and will bring about a general reformation. The mythical agents of its spread are the R.C. Brothers [R.C. = Rosicrucian], devoutly evangelical. Their religious faith seems closely connected with their alchemical philosophy, which has nothing to do with 'ungodly and accursed gold making', for the riches which Father Rosencreutz offers are spiritual; 'He doth not rejoice that he can make gold but is glad that he seeth the Heavens open, and the angels of God ascending and descending, and his name written in the Book of Life.[5]

The relevance of the manifestos lies in their influence on philosophers and scientists all over Europe. That an actual Rosicrucian Brotherhood existed is, in fact, very doubtful, as no evidence as to who they were or where they lived has been found or verified by scholars. Many European thinkers read the tracts and then searched for the source in vain. They could receive no reply to their enquiries. Perhaps there are still hidden sources and more light could be shed on the exact intent of the manifestos. The importance of Rosicrucian ideas and influences is that they were widespread over several cultures simultaneously and with varying results.

Scholars both in England and other European cultures were branded Rosicrucians if they so much as espoused any of the views or ideas contained in the manifestos, in whatever form. This happened to Robert Fludd who was accused of being a defender of the Rosicrucian Brotherhood, due to two of his works which expressed admiration for their ideas and aims. These works had, as it happened, been his own attempt to contact the writers of the manifestos, and his desire to contribute to their work. He firmly believed that they did exist, although he admitted he had never met one of them. What is possibly more important for the spread of ideas is that Fludd's books were published by the De Bry firm in Oppenheim which also published the works of Michael Maier, an important alchemical writer of the same period. It is often said that the two men influenced each other, since both were Paracelsian physicians. Fludd was mostly influenced by Paracelsist alchemy and by John Dee, as well as the Renaissance tradition of Magia and Cabala; and Maier was swayed by the influences he received at the court of Rudloph II at Prague, during the period that he was appointed physician.

As Frances Yates has analysed in great depth, it is no accident that these manifestos appeared precisely during the reign of Frederick and Elizabeth of the Palatinate; and ended abruptly with the overthrow of their principality by Hapsburg forces in 1620. No more Rosicrucian manifestos appeared after this date. They can therefore, also, be seen as having very specific political intent, to foster an aspect of the Protestant reformation, its impulse to renew 'enlightened' attempts at learning. The coupling of this particular aspect of Protestantism with alchemical and Christian symbolism and allegory is of great fascination, as the interest in medicine, healing, spiritual alchemical transformation, Christian symbolism and a keen insistence on the coming of a new age of thought permeates the entire Rosicrucian attempt in those few years. This left an indelible influence on many European thinkers, from scientists to medical men, artists and philosophers.

The actual political failure of the Elector of the Palatinate to become the spearhead and focal point of this intellectual and social renewal is also very interesting in the light of what then became the dominant countering force in Heidelberg and other major European seats of learning. The Thirty Years War being no mean or light experience, much of the impulse disseminated to France, the Lowlands, Britain, and many other countries.

The manifestos had created a great stir and were reprinted to fulfil an ever increasing demand. The printed manifesto or book was becoming more widely read, although one must not forget that, even so, very few were yet able to read. But, with the spread of books, learning via texts became more widespread, and in the language of each country not just in Latin, although the majority of learned texts were still in Latin.

The first Rosicrucian manifestos were clearly influenced by John Dee.

John Dee personified the Renaissance magus in his fullest dignity (though in a rather extreme form since he came so late in time). Pico Della Mirandola describes the power of the magus in the *Oration on the Dignity of Man*. 'O supreme generosity of God the Father, O highest and most marvellous felicity of man! To him is granted to have whatever he chooses, to be whatever he wills. Beasts as soon as they are born (so says Lucilius) bring with them from their mother's womb all things they will ever possess. Spiritual beings, either from the beginning or soon thereafter, become what they are to be for ever and ever. On man when he came into life the Father conferred seeds of all kinds and the germs of every way of life. Whatever seeds each man cultivates will grow to maturity and bear in him their own fruit. If they be vegative, he will be like a plant. If sensitive, he will become brutish. If rational, he will grow into a heavenly being. If intellectual, he will be an angel and the son of God. And if, happy in the lot of no created thing, he withdraws into the centre of his own unity, made one with God, in the solitary darkness of God, who is set above all things, shall surpass them all.'

This was the spirit of the Renaissance Hermetic tradition that began with Ficino – to give man in his power, his intellectual capacity, his beauty, a place beside God. The relationship between God and man was defined in a new and revolutionary way and was to have far reaching results.[6]

The other figure mentioned earlier, Michael Maier, performed a most interesting function in this cross-fertilization of cultures and ideas which manifested as the Rosicrucian philosophy of the early seventeenth century. He, too, was a Paracelsian physician, dedicated to the spiritual and contemplative-religious aspect of alchemy. He often served as a bridge between England, Prague and the Palatinate. His contemplations, and those of Robert Fludd, published by the De Bry publishing firm in Oppenheim, were perhaps the most full and explicit of the 'Rosicrucian' texts.

Both men's works were amply and beautifully illustrated with engravings of symbolic-alchemical images. Those of Michael Maier were allegorical, while those of Fludd were more mathematical and hierarchical, dealing mainly with the microcosm-macrocosm. Many of the engravings for their books were executed by the same engraver, Lucas Jennis; both writers, especially Fludd, gave specific instructions on the images. These were all worthy of attention and the famous engravings of Maier's *Atalanta Fugiens* will be familiar to some. Powerful they certainly are and, in the case of this particular book, each image is accompanied by a musical equivalent. These are perhaps some of the most impressive alchemical texts, exposing the full tenor of the influences mentioned above: Dee, Paracelsus, the earlier neo-Platonic ideas. Giordano Bruno may have influenced Maier's thinking, also, since Bruno had left his mark on various groups of Protestants during his brief stay in Germany at the end of the sixteenth century.

Maier's involvement as appointed physician with the court at Prague and the court of the Palatinate, as well as the Landgrave of Hesse, allowed him to have access to what may have been the seat of the Rosicrucian Brotherhood. His frequent travelling between Heidelberg, Prague and England indicated a reciprocity of ideas and aims.

How do Bacon and Newton fit into this tapestry of ideas? In what way do these enormous changes in ideas relate to the change taking place in medicine? Unless we understand the undercurrents of philosophical ideas and the way in which European cultures fed and influenced each other via their thinkers, we cannot understand the change taking place in medical practice or the social mores, reflecting these changes, which often determined the choices for specific uses of medicine. The role of the physician, also, can better be understood in this framework of change. Reaction and counter-reaction always seem to camouflage what is often the natural transformation of ideas and practice. The great religious changes sweeping across Europe in the seventeenth century had also a deep and devastating effect.

That the Hermetic tradition was very much alive, while the more mechanical tools of research were developing, is no accident. Throughout the seventeenth century mechanical tools of research were being invented, the microscope being only one of many. Astronomers were discovering new relationships between the stars and the earth, and whole vistas were opening into the nature of man's concept of his physical reality.

Francis Bacon (1561–1626) is often regarded as the true mind behind the beginnings of the 'real' scientific empiricism. It is very interesting to note that Bacon's important publications began in 1605 with *The Advancement of Learning*, during the reign of James I and prior to the publication of the Rosicrucian manifestos. His next publications, however, including the important *Novum Organum* (1620) were contemporaneous with the Rosicrucian outpourings. Bacon was a very different man, indeed, to the men already discussed. He was fully aware of James I's antagonism to, and fear of, anything that might tell of magic, alchemy or the hermetic vein of thought. Shortly before Bacon's publication of *The Advancement of Learning*, Dee's work had been publicly repudiated by James I. Thus, Bacon proceeded carefully; he advanced to powerful public office. Europe and England were entering the fiercest stage of the witch-hunting and persecution of ideas antagonistic to the power of the Church. Protestant countries were the fiercest in their persecution.

Bacon's main goal was to make a clear plan for the study and clarification of all the sciences. His ideals for learning were not at all dissimilar to the Rosicrucian ideals, although his emphasis was in a different area. A new restoration of great learning, the Great Instauration or *Magna Instauratio* was envisaged by Bacon as his most important work. In it he laid down the ways by which learning must proceed, by ridding itself of the 'bane' of Aristotelian thought and by examining the reality of nature and things as clearly and pragmatically as possible.

In the first section of *The Advancement of Learning,* while discussing the largely theological reasons why knowledge and the acquisition of learning and knowledge had been considered heretical or atheistic, that is, leading men away from God, Bacon makes the following comments:

To this we answer, I. It was not pure knowledge of nature, by the light whereof man gave names to all the creatures in Paradise, agreeable to their natures, that occasioned the fall; but the proud knowledge of good and evil, with an intent in man to give Law to himself, and depend no more on God. II. Nor can any quantity of natural knowledge puff up the mind; for nothing fills, much less distends the Soul, but God. Whence as Solomon declares: 'That the eye is not satisfied with seeing, nor

60

can the ear with hearing; so knowledge itself he says, God hath made all things beautiful in their seasons; also he hath placed the world in man's heart; yet cannot man find out the work which God worketh from the beginning to the end'; hereby declaring plainly that God has framed the mind like a glass, capable of the image of the universe, and desirous to receive it as the eye to receive light; and thus it is not only pleased with the variety and vissicitudes of things, but also endeavours to find out the laws they observe in their changes and alterations. And if such be the extent of the mind, there is no danger of filling it with any quantity of knowledge. But it is merely from its quality when taken without the true corrections, that knowledge has somewhat of venom or malignity.... The corrective which renders it sovereign is charity, for according to St. Paul: 'knowledge puffeth up, but charity buildeth.'[7]

Bacon's contribution may very well have reached the notice of thinkers in the Palatinate. And yet we cannot say that Bacon was a Rosicrucian, as such, although he had a great interest in the Hermetic-alchemical tradition. Frances Yates points out:

Recent scholarship has made it abundantly clear that the old view of Bacon as a modern scientific observer and experimentalist emerging out of a superstitious past is no longer valid. In his book on Bacon, Paolo Rossi (*Francis Bacon, From Magic to Science*, London 1968), has shown that it was out of the Hermetic tradition that Bacon emerged, out of the Magia and Cabala of the Renaissance as it had reached him via the natural magicians. Bacon's view of the future of science was not that of progress in a straight line. His great instauration of science was directed towards a return to the state of Adam before the Fall, a state of pure and sinless contact with nature and knowledge of her powers. This was the view of scientific progress, a progress back towards Adam, held by Cornelius Agrippa, the author of the influential Renaissance textbook of occult sciences. Amongst the subjects he reviews in his survey of learning are natural magic; astrology, of which he seeks a reformed version; alchemy, by which he was profoundly influenced; fascination, the tool of the magician, and other themes which those interested in drawing out the modern side of Bacon have set aside as unimportant.[8]

Bacon, however, separated himself from thinkers such as Fludd, as it was not politic to align with such overt 'Hermetic' thinking, especially that of Fludd's philosophical emphasis on the macrocosm-microcosm. Indeed, Bacon was not fully in accord with this idea. Not until the publication of *The New Atlantis* does Bacon show his vision of the future of 'enlightened' learning, equally as idealistic as, and similar to, the Rosicrucian manifestos, even in some of its symbolism and allegory. This, an undated manuscript, found amongst Bacon's unpublished works, was published a year after his death in 1627. In the midst of this huge upsurge of thinking and innovation in the seventeenth century, Bacon's references, in no way, would have been overlooked.

It is commonly thought that Bacon's work led directly to the formation of the Royal Society, in the hands of Ashmole and others. The Society was founded in order to create an arena for the pursuit of scientific research and knowledge, as well as provide a forum for the exchange of ideas and learning and thus enable scholars to perform a useful role in society.

Sir Isaac Newton (1642–1727), without doubt one of the greatest scientific minds of the seventeenth century, was also linked to the Rosicrucian tradition. In no time at all the Royal Society departed from the influence of Bacon and became dominated by the great mind of Newton. By 1686, with the publication of his *Principia*, produced after twenty years of intensive work, Newton created a huge stir in the minds of European scholars and scientists.

The *Principia* was the great work in which Newton expounded his accurately formulated mathematical theory of gravitation as well as his laws on the workings of nature. Until this century, Newton's enormous contribution has largely been viewed as that positing a completely mechanical system of the workings of nature and the universe. He had, however, a considerable interest in both theology and alchemy. The joining of Newton the mathematician and Newton the mystic is too important to overlook, especialiy in the philosophical context of the seventeenth century. He left unpublished more papers on theology and alchemy than were ever published on science.

According to the writings of his secretary at Cambridge, where he was Professor of Mathematics for many years, he spent hours closeted in his laboratory pursuing the finer experiments of his work on metallurgy and other related areas; for this prowess he was appointed Master of the Mint in 1699.

Prominent in Newton's library were works on alchemy, as well as English translations of the Rosicrucian manifestos; and of prime interest to him was Ashmole's *Theatrum Chemicum Brittanicum*, an anthology of British alchemical writings. In this work Ashmole attempted to keep alive the tradition connected with the Rosicrucian impulse.

Another great fascination for Newton was the work of the German mystic, Jakob Bohme, to the extent that he had lovingly copied out in his own hand large passages from Bohme's work. One can see that the many strains of seventeenth-century thought met in Newton's questing mind and deep intellectual enquiry into the plan of the earth and stars; these influences ranged from Galileo's discoveries, through Kepler's laws, Bohme's theology and his own deep love of alchemical pursuits. The development of mathematics was also part of this tradition. It stemmed from Dee and others and, to a certain extent, culminated in the seventeenth century in Newton's brilliant synthesis of the mathematical logic in the gravitational nature of the relationship of the planets and stars to the earth, as well as the function of magnetic attraction and repulsion in terms of gravity on the earth itself. Frances Yates comments:

> The more recent Newton scholarship has emphasized the Renaissance type of thinking at the back of Newton's scientific efforts, his belief in the tradition of ancient wisdom concealed in myth, and his confidence that he had himself discovered the true philosophy behind mythology.[9]

Again, we can see that the interpretation of Newton's work has often been one-sided. A man's work must be seen as a totality, in the context of the deep undercurrents of his time. Here we see a joining of what have often been posited as antitheses to each other: the spiritual-alchemical-religious and the mechanical-scientific. Intermingled, they created a startling and innovative synthesis, opening new thresholds of discovery.

As Christopher Hill pointed out in his essay on 'Newton and his Society':

> It is no more possible to treat the history of Science as something uncontaminated by the world in which the scientists lived than it is to write the history of, say, philosophy or literature or the English constitution in isolation from the societies which gave birth to them.[10]

Great debate, refutation and scepticism abounded for a lengthy period over Newton's theories. The subject of his work is vast and complex, but to give a small glimpse of how Newton himself saw his philosophy let us quote briefly from the *Principia*. In this passage we can clearly see the joining of both the vitalist and the mechanical in his outlook.

> And now we might add something concerning a certain most subtle spirit which pervades and hides in all gross bodies; by the force and action of which spirit the particles of bodies attract one another at near distances, and cohere if contiguous; and electric bodies operate to greater distances, as well repelling as attracting the neighbouring corpuscles; and light is emitted, reflected, refracted, inflected, and heats bodies; and all sensation is excited, and the member of animal bodies move at the command of the will, namely by the vibrations of this spirit, mutually propagated along the solid filaments of the nerves, from the outward organs of sense to the brain, and from the brain into the muscles. But these are things that cannot be explained in few words, nor are we furnished with the sufficiency of experiments required to an accurate determination and demonstration of the laws by which this electric and elastic spirit operates.[11]

Of himself and his achievements, Newton wrote:

> I do not know what I may appear to the world; but to myself I seem to have been only like a boy playing on the seashore, and

diverting myself in now and then finding a smoother pebble or a prettier shell than ordinary, while the great ocean of truth lay undiscovered before me.[12]

Looking further ahead at the influence of these discoveries, it is interesting to note Arthur Koestler's comments in his book, *The Sleepwalkers*. In summing up the new scientific vistas of the period, especially those of physics, he comments on the process as a 'vanishing act' in the seeming divorce between science and religion. 'Freed from mystical ballast, science could sail ahead at breathtaking speed to its conquest of new lands beyond every dream.'[13] Yet, Koestler also points to a loss in 'progress', a distinct polarity:

> Each advance in physical theory, with its rich technological harvest, was bought by a loss in intelligibility. These losses on the intellectual balance sheet, however, were much less in evidence than the spectacular gains; they were light-heartedly accepted as passing clouds which the next advance would dissolve. The seriousness of the impasse became only apparent in the second quarter of this century, and then only to the more philosophically minded among scientists, who had retained a certain immunity against what we might call the new scholasticism of theoretical physics.[14]

This insight is of interest here, as a parting of the ways became more evident by the eighteenth century. This subtle separation between religion, especially described here in an idealistic form, and science, did indeed become more and more apparent.

We can now start to examine the impact that both scientific discoveries and the Rosicrucian tradition had on the development of European medicine at the end of the seventeenth, and beginning of the eighteenth, centuries.

As Mircea Eliade so lucidly put it in his last volume of *A History of Religious Ideas*:

> In its spectacular flight, 'modern science' has ignored, or rejected, the heritage of Hermeticism. Or to put it differently,

the triumph of Newtonian mechanics has ended up by annihilating its own scientific ideal. In effect, Newton and his contemporaries expected a different type of scientific revolution. In prolonging and developing the hopes and objectives (the first among these being the redemption of Nature) of the neo-alchemist of the Renaissance, minds as different as those of Paracelsus, John Dee, Comenius, J.V. Andrae, Fludd, and Newton saw in alchemy the model for a no less ambitious enterprise: the perfection of man by a new method of know-ledge.... This type of 'knowledge', dreamed of and partially elaborated in the eighteenth century, represents the last enterprise of Christian Europe that was undertaken with the aim of obtaining 'total knowledge'.[15]

Notes – Chapter 4

1. Frances Yates, *The Rosicrucian Enlightenment*, London, Paladin, 1975, p.11.
2. Peter French, *John Dee, the World of an Elizabethan Magus*, London, Routledge, Kegan Paul, 1984, p.22.
3. John Dee, *Heptarchia Mystica,* Aquarian Press, 1986, pp. 13–14.
4. French, op. cit.
5. Yates, op. cit., p. 75.
6. French, op. cit., pp. 63–4.
7. Francis Bacon, *The Advancement of Learning,* New York, Willey Book Co., 1900, p. 3.
8. F. Yates, op. cit., pp. 156–7.
9. ibid., pp. 247–8.
10. Christopher Hill, 'Newton and His Society', *The Annus Mirabilis of Sir Isaac Newton 1666–1966*, Cambridge Mass. & London, MIT Press, 1970.
11. Isaac Newton, *Principia*, p. 547.
12. Newton, *Andriade*, p. 131.
13. Arthur Koestler, *The Sleepwalkers. A History of Man's Changing Vision of the Universe* London, Pelican Books, 1968, p. 539.
14. ibid., p. 540.
15. Mircea Eliade, *A History of Religious Ideas*, vol. 3, Chicago, University of Chicago Press, 1985 p. 261.

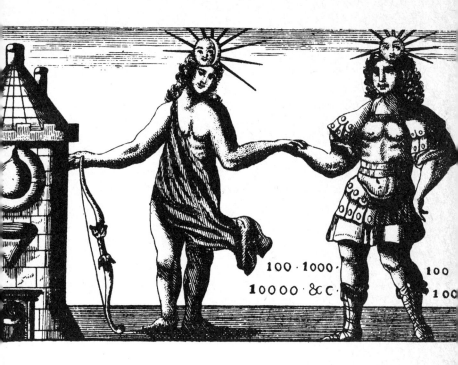

100 · 1000 ·   100
10000 · &c ·   100

5   Medicine and the Enlightenment

'I perceive' said the Countess, 'Philosophy is now become very mechanical.'

'So mechanical' said I, 'that I fear we shall quickly be ashamed of it; they will have the world be great, what a watch is in little; which is very regular, and depends only upon the just disposing of the several parts of the movement. But pray tell me, Madam, had you not formerly a more sublime idea of the universe?'

Fontenelle, *Plurality of Worlds*

At the end of the seventeenth, and the beginning of the eighteenth, centuries the rise of mechanical thinking became evident. This system conceived of man and the universe as a magnificent machine, made of wondrous efficient parts, created by God, of course, but a marvel in its perfect, machine-like, determinable parts; a precision instrument.

As the great impetus to discover reality proceeded via the many 'scientific' breakthroughs and discoveries about the nature of the earth, its relationship to the stars, to movement, gravity, geometric and mathematical logic so, too, came into question the nature of God's role and man's role in relation to divine intervention or revelation. A 'miracle' became a debatable fact, as did the perfection of the scriptures or even the notion of the 'fall' of Adam and Eve. The eighteenth century saw the dawning of an age of greater scepticism, agnosticism and divergence from religion; yet there was also a growth of scattered groupings within the major religions, dependent on an overall view of rationality and a belief that all facts could, and should, be a matter of logical deduction. A new, yet often demeaning, scientific and mathematical model of man in his world was abroad with many far-reaching consequences, both positive and negative.

The Age of Reason is the name so often given to the eighteenth century. During this Age of Reason devastating epidemic disease was rife: smallpox which killed large numbers throughout Europe: bubonic plague and also influenza. There were high rates of infant mortality and death of the mother in childbirth. The average age of man, according to Voltaire, was twenty-two, if he was a lucky man.

The grand monarchs reigned supreme throughout most of that century. The first voyages to countries later to become colonies of the European nations, began with traders and missionaries to the Far and Middle East and to other 'undiscovered' parts of the globe. 'The nobel savage' was a new and disturbing factor to the European mind, an indication that other cultures and other races had long evolved men and women of wisdom outside the influence of Christianity or the cradle of the West. These other cultures also had radically different methods of dealing with health.

China, especially, was a revelation to European travellers, missionaries and discoverers alike. The Chinese, as well as the Turks, had given 'vaccinations' for a very long time. Such a practice, both commonplace and accepted, utilized droplets of the disease serum by entering them into the blood system with small needles in the skin, as protection against the disease.

This was the age, too, of Bach, Haydn and, later, Mozart, the great courts fostering some of the greatest European music. There was consolidation of power in the growing nation states, a developing commerce and a recovery from the tumult of the seventeenth century; yet, this period led to two revolutions: the French and the American (1789–95 and 1775–85).

Despite the fact that disease was rampant and longevity rare, populations were growing. Internal sanitation was almost non-existent. Insanity was still treated as a scourge on humanity, the 'mad' in chains being locked away from the light of day to be observed by a curious and abusive public on ceremonious occasions. People could be locked away on any pretext and the level of brutality was terrible in institutions of supposed charity.

Meanwhile, the ill were leeched, bloodlet, purged and treated by a variety of 'learned' doctors who ranged from the few who were endowed with some stature to the majority of bewigged, swaying, socially acceptable 'doctors', administering the medical practices and medicines of the age.

Voltaire had two diverse ways of describing the state of medicine during his lifetime: 'Out of every hundred physicians ninety-eight are charlatans.' And, speaking of an ideal physician, he comments, 'Men who are occupied in the restoration of health to other men, by joint exercises of skill and humanity, are above all the great men of the earth. They even partake of divinity, since to preserve and to renew is almost as noble as to create.'[1]

How then was medicine being practised, and how was medical and scientific knowledge and discovery evolving over the century into which Hahnemann was born? Not only had iatrochemistry continued to exist in its fragmentary way, but other influences which had their roots in the preceeding century caused further divisions. Mechanical thinkers in the scientific and medical fields were divided into two groups: the iatromathematicians and the iatromechanists. We have looked briefly at the effect Bacon's and Newton's work had on the entire scientific world. Now we will examine Descartes' role in formulating theories which were also to have an enormous effect.

René Descartes (1596–1650) is possibly best known for his work, *Discourse on Method* (1637). One of his main aims was to sweep away the errors of the past, a common concern of many of the thinkers previously considered, and to seek and discover the importance of mathematics by application of algebra and geometry. Within this construct was the well-known Cartesian method of doubt. In his survey of how the world came into being by physical laws, he proposed a mechanical explanation at almost all points, from astronomy to animals and man in particular. He describes the human body 'as a machine made by the hands of God, which is incomparably better arranged and adequate to movements more admirable than is any machine of human invention'.[2]

Greatly influenced by Galileo and by Harvey's discoveries, Descartes was able to define the laws of inertia (momentum = quantity of matter X its velocity). Galileo had only come close to this and had been seen as an heretical force by the Catholic Church. Galileo's trial took place in 1633 and, from then on, Descartes took great care not to antagonize the Church. This aspect of Descartes's makeup may have influenced his formulations of scientific and metaphysical theories, for he had no desire to be a martyr. He remained in fear of contradicting the Church's authority; this fear created a dualism that is present throughout his work. He had to find room in his system of thought for two entirely separate worlds: a model of a purely mechanical world, on the one hand, to a certain extent the basis of modern materialism and, on the other hand, a conception of the Soul as separate from the body, a concept of God as separate from the world.

Descartes rejected the existence of atoms, a theory put forth in his lifetime by Boyle and others. He evolved, however, a theory of vortices into which all particles of matter were collected. Nevertheless, he did base many of his theories on a notion of particles in matter. Primarily, having discovered the laws of vision as being geometric in nature, he made an assumption that all knowledge of the body could be submitted to mathematical logic and examination.

Descartes also offered another description of the human body, saying it is

> but a statue, an earthen machine formed intentionally by God . . . not only does he give it externally the shapes and colours of all parts of our bodies; He also places inside it all the pieces required to make it walk, eat, breathe, and imitate whichever of our own functions can be imagined to proceed from mere matter and to depend entirely on the arrangement of our organs.[3]

At the very base of his method was his insistence on not deducing and perceiving the particular from the universal but, rather, to proceed from the universal to the particular. He believed that an individual who followed his method accurately could attain to the whole of human knowledge via the perfection, as he saw it, of mathematics.

His mathematical knowledge and understanding was enormous. Errors in his thinking seemed to occur when he applied this purely mathematical logic to other fields that commanded his interest. In defining how man should reason and perceive truth, Descartes made a distinction between reason by mathematical deduction and either perception or imagination. The latter two he saw as bearing no fruit in the direction of knowledge; furthermore, they were often a hindrance in attaining it. Only clear vision of the intellect gives knowledge, according to Descartes's way of thinking; he called this 'intuition'.

> By *intuition* I understand, not the fluctuating testimony of the senses, nor the misleading judgement that proceeds from the blending constructions of the imagination, but the conception which an unclouded and attentive mind gives us so readily and distinctly that we are wholly freed from doubt about that which we understand. Or what comes to the same thing, intuition is the undoubting conception of an unclouded and attentive mind, and springs from the light of reason alone; it is more certain than deduction itself, in that it is simpler, though deduction cannot by us be erroneously conducted.[4]

The stark division between mind and body is surmised to have taken place through Descartes and his influence on European ideas. Out of a century riddled with war, death and pestilence, two men in particular, Newton and Descartes, in quite different ways, had a broad and momentous influence in determining what was to become the evolved 'modern' scientific method. Behind these men's work lay Galileo's struggle and success in putting the Aristotelian world to the test, and opening radically new vistas in understanding matter, force, the functioning of space and bodies and the many relationships between the earth and the stars.

The reign of man's desire to control nature, as opposed to being at unity with nature, was slowly but surely entering into

73

the domain of most fields of enquiry; this was particularly so in the sciences and had an overwhelming influence on medicine and its development.

There were numerous philosophers, thinkers, scientists and pioneers in this period who need not be discussed here, as the task at hand is to understand the development and changes in the medical art. The shift in emphasis on different forms of perception was to change the face of medical enquiry, theory and practice. Despite these great changes in scientific discovery, and sometimes because of them, medicine underwent a number of strange and tumultuous events in the eighteenth century, not finding its feet in a secure method or outlook, although some of its participants may have believed that they had found the absolute answers.

As the century progressed an additional confusion of ideas entered the arena. Discoveries made about the body, by way of closer scrutiny of its anatomical properties, were becoming more acceptable. The body considered as an excellent machine took more dominance as an idea and structure in which to perceive illness while, at the same time, many diverse medical philosophies and practices existed in various European nations.

The debate between the 'vitalist' and mechanical vision of man was rife throughout this period and, even within this debate, varying methods of diagnosis and treatment were employed. A more confused period for a physician could hardly have existed despite the growing 'security' of ideas of a burgeoning enlightenment and a supposed concern for the welfare of man on a social level. For some, the more accepted medical ideas were considered the peak of the evolution of thought in that area; for others, constant questioning continued. Then, too, the growth of new forms of philosophical enquiry and 'natural philosophy' also had their influences on medical ideas.

One of the more influential physicians of the earlier part of this period, in one area of thought, the vitalist, was George Ernest Stahl (1660–1734). The majority of seventeenth- and eighteenth-century doctors had followed in the footsteps of the new Cartesian world view, incorporating these ideas into the varying groups of iatromechanists, iatrochemists and iatro-mathematicians. At this stage the majority of iatrochemists had combined their changing chemical views with the newer mechanical hypotheses and discoveries in physics and anatomy. Unlike Stahl's contemporaries, Boerhaave, Hoffman, Baglivi and others of the more mechanical schools, Stahl rejected Descartes almost outright. In his view the Cartesian system suppressed an understanding of all forms of life which were pressed into concepts of organized matter, with little or no reference to outer forces, to Divinity, or to the Soul; thus all relationship was conceptualized as being of a purely mechanical nature.

Stahl, however, conceived a theory of 'animism' which, to a certain extent, dominated areas of medicine at that time, just as his theory of 'phlogiston', the principal of combustibility, dominated chemistry until it either dissipated in the nineteenth century or was superceded by other chemical discoveries.

At the start of his career Stahl had been influenced by Boerhaave, Hoffman and Baglivi. Hoffman brought him to the University of Halle in 1694 where Stahl became the Professor of Pathology, Physiology, Pharmacology, Chemistry and Botany. They were later estranged when their views diverged. Stahl remained at the University until 1716 when he became physician to the King of Prussia, Frederick William I, in Berlin, until Stahl's death in 1734.

What is interesting about Stahl's work, theories and practice was his concept of the *Anima Sensitiva*, also called by him and his followers the 'Reasonable Soul'. This he saw as the only governing form of the corporeal economy of man. The curative power of man he also saw as residing in the Soul (*Anima*). Stahl also believed that the *Anima* could behave independently from the body, that is, with its own intrinsic intelligence. Sickness was the effort of the Anima to re-establish the normal tone, operation and harmony of disordered organs.

This was a purely vitalistic approach to man, the cure of illness and the maintenance of health. Stahl's theories were adopted by the large and important medical school in Montpellier and also formed the philosophical basis of medicine in the Paris school of medicine. Between these two schools differences did exist. In Montpellier there was a more 'animistic' view, while the Paris school incorporated an understanding of dynamism within the concept of mechanical medicine. Stahl's influence continued for a very long time indeed. In Montpellier, the 'animistic' concept saw the principal of life as the 'Vital Force', which they believed to be the power which organizes and supports the whole of matter, as distinguished from physical forces, either mechanical or chemical.

And yet, when one looks more closely at Stahl's work, and the work and writings of those working alongside him and after him in these two schools, one can see many contradictions. Mainly, he seemed to concentrate a great deal on theory and not on methods or practical use of medicines. Thus, many different methods of practice emerged that could, potentially, be fitted into his theoretical structure. Stahl was adamantly opposed to the current practice of the use of large doses of medicine or the administration of quantities of different medicines simultaneously. As he wrote:

Cleansing the pharmacy of our times is more than the labour of Hercules who undertook to cleanse the Augean stables. Here it is a stable, but not of horses, but of asses. What honest practitioner who is skillful and serious does not realize that the modern pharmacopoepia abounds in superfluous, imprudent, uncertain, absurdly compounded, and dangerous remedies bequeathed to us by the ancients as well as by the Greek and Arab pharmocologists. They have been further sullied by the audacious and imprudent lies of charlatans, hawkers at fairs, charcoal sellers, barbers, and stupid empirics and accompanied by their ... comments resounding in superlatives, are so praised as to make those who sell them to the public at the fairs and markets, together with their ... eulogies, rightly ridiculous. Certainly these latter remedies are piles of ass ... which no river can ever wash away.[5]

Stahl maintained that the true source of medical knowledge was the observation of the visible acts of the *Anima*. He wrote,

'Everything in medicine is based on clinical practice and on precise observation of the facts furnished us by experience.'[6]

To quote from Harris Coulter's *Divided Legacy*:

> Stahl did not define or classify these procedures of the 'anima', and did not create an elaborate doctrine of therapeutic intervention, leaving these two points to his followers for solution.
>
> The first was attached dramatically by Francois Bossier de la Croix de Sauvages (1706–1767) who introduced the Stahlian doctrine to Montpellier. An acute mathematician and Iatro-mechanist who felt that his mechanically conceived organism needed a motivating force, Sauvages followed the suggestions made by Sydenham and Baglivi and described in symptomatic terms all the illnesses and diseases known to medicine at that time – a total of about 2500. These patterns combined the impact of the morbific stimulus and the reaction of the 'anima'. Sauvages' therapeutics, however, remained conventional and eclectic.
>
> He was followed by Theophile Bordeu, a more subtle and realistic thinker and one of the great figures of French medical history.... Bordeu aligned the 'anima' more closely with the Hippocratic 'physis' clothing it with the biological and physiological concepts developed by his contemporaries while retaining its purposiveness and spontaneity. This led to an original and valuable interpretation of the glandular system (making him a pioneer of endocronology) and an understanding of the voluntary and sympathetic nervous systems. But his pharmacology, like that of Stahl, was rudimentary.
>
> The final apotheosis of Animism in Montpellier, lasting through the nineteenth century, was that of Paul-Joseph Barthez (1754–1806).[7]

According to Stahl the physical body exists for the sake of the *Anima* and was thus its instrument. The presence of the *Anima* thus distinguishes the body from being only a mass of chemicals or a piece of machinery.

Stahl ascribed all the movements of the body to the *Anima* which, among its other functions, reacts to external morbific influences. The number of such reactions were infinite. Sauvages curtailed this freedom of the *Anima*, dividing the organism into an area subject to the *Anima* directly and a second area which, while ultimately dynamized by the *Anima*, functions as a hydraulic machine. The *Anima* possesses 'animate forces', and the organism-as-hydraulic machine functions through its 'inanimate forces' which follow the ordinary laws of physics and chemistry.[8]

Stahl's more unified image of illness and the vital principle was thus reduced to a divided analysis. What had started as a model based on observation and experience became, with Sauvages's work, a method which looked reductively at disease classes.

Meanwhile, in Scotland, William Cullen (1710–90) and his student, John Brown (1735–88) were to have a broad influence over late eighteenth- and early nineteenth-century medicine throughout Europe. Cullen's work shaped the views of many generations of students and was considered the pinnacle of eighteenth-century medical thinking. Cullen had been trained in the system of Boerhaave, based largely on humoralism. Cullen, however, was more concerned with solids and their motions. He developed an entire doctrine on the definition of life as 'excitement of the nervous system'. Brown took this one step further to say that life *is* excitability, a quality which follows its own laws. He posited that 'Health consists in a balance between the inherant "excitability" and the internal or external "exciting powers".[9]

In describing the role of excitement and the nervous system, Cullen states, 'Life, so far as it is corporeal, we suppose to consist in the excitement of the nervous system, and especially of the brain, which unites the different parts and forms them into a whole.'[10]

His treatment of disease was always with contraries. Reactions in the blood system were moderated by bloodletting, acids, neutral salts, purges, sedatives and exercise. 'Spasms' were eliminated by antispasmodics such as opium and camphor, blistering and warm baths. Debility or weakness was restored by tonics and stimulants.

Brown divided disease into two forms, 'asthenic' (diseases of 'direct debility' or 'want of irritation') and 'sthenic' (diseases of 'indirect debility' or too much irritation). The first he treated with remedies which supported 'excitement', such as the application of heat, roast beef, opium, exercise, whisky, wines and spirits. The 'sthenic' disease required a lowering treatment, such as bleeding, application of cold, vomiting, sweating and a starvation diet. Brown simplified to such an extent that he saw very little difference between any patients and any diseases:

Instead of the infinite differences of habits and temperament, I have found every individual precisely the same as every other. Whatever produces the gout in one will produce it in another prepared to receive its influence. And whatever cures it in anyone, cures it also in every other; and so forth with respect to every other disease. The deeper we explore the works of nature, the more shall we be convinced of this wonderful simplicity.[11]

He later comments.

Such is the simplicity to which medicine is thus reduced that when a physician comes to the bedside of a patient, he has only three things to settle in his mind. First, whether the disease be general, whether it is sthenic or asthenic; thirdly, what is its degree? When once he has satisfied himself in these points, all that remains for him to do is to form his indications or general view of the plan of cure and carry that into execution by the administration of proper remedies.[12]

Since both Cullen's and, especially, Brown's medical methods swept across the European medical world in the late eighteenth and early nineteenth centuries, the simplification of Brown's methods and the authority of Cullen were both widely acknowledged in Germany. Hahnemann could hardly have remained unaware of this.

New authorities in medicine seemed to rise and fall quite rapidly at this time – and much confusion abounded. These were the forms of medicine Hahnemann would have encountered as a student, a scholar and a young medical practitioner. It is not surprising, as we shall see, that he questioned all established precepts. When writing about the state of medicine in Germany as it neared the nineteenth century, the Professor of Clinical Medicine at Mainz noted, in 1812, that the interests of the medical profession kept changing rapidly and almost vainly.

I know a physician who at one time adopted the heating and sweating method. How much *essentia alexipharmica, mistura simplex* and *composita Stahlii* did he not daily prescribe! He was also a great partisan of bleeding, and I do not doubt that he often counteracted the baneful effects of his heating remedies and vice versa. But the triumverate of Boerhaave, Stahl and Fr. Hoffman was drawing to an end. Tissot became the leading authority. Our practitioners now advocated the cooling method. Tamarinds, cream of tartar, saltpetre, oxymel, and barley water were his favourite remedies. He forbade healthy people to smoke, because Tissot had asserted that all tobacco-smokers must die in their prime of apoplexy. When Stoll became the leading authority among physicians, we find tartar emetic and ipecac in most of their prescriptions. They were, of course, devoted to the administration of clysters when Kampt was in vogue. [Clysters were made from a combination of eleven or twelve medicines.] C.L. Hoffman was called to occupy the place that had been held by this physician. Accustomed to follow the spirit of the age, they now exaggerated what this great thinker taught concerning antiseptic remedies. How can fashionable practitioners understand the meaning of an author? Enough; our physicians did not observe how the functions of their patients were carried on, in order to ascertain how far these were injurious or advantageous to the maintenance of the body, but they proceeded forthwith to cure every disease by means of antiseptics. A few years later Brown became dictator in medicine, and 'Methodism' ruled the fashion. Our practitioners now called those physicians who devoted themselves to remedy vices in the fluids of the body, or to procure evacuation of depraved humours, murderers; for to believe in such vices showed the greatest ignorance. Their practice was summed up in four words – sthenia, asthenia, sthenic influence, asthenic vices. Very few of their prescriptions were without naptha, laudanum, ether, musk, or sal-ammoniac. They were now as much in favour of wine, brandy, and meat diet, as they had been against them at the time when Tissot was the ruling deity. Now they returned to purging in order to cure local affections, and tried to unite all these different modes of treatment. Therefore, they now refused to be called Brownians, and insisted upon being called eclectics.[13]

From this description of just how unstable medical views were at the end of the eighteenth century and the turn of the nineteenth, we can ascertain how perturbing this must have been to a young medical man, especially one as enquiring as Hahnemann. We have had a glimpse of the many medical methods that emerged in the eighteenth century, all with varying methodology and emphasis. Edward Jenner had introduced the use of innoculation against smallpox. Lavoisier had made great strides in chemistry. More and more research done into the particular and the mechanical and, yet, a complete model for medical practice had not been found.

In this context let us take a look at Hahnemann, his work and the inception of homoeopathic medicine.

Notes – Chapter 5

1.   Fontenelle, *Plurality of Worlds*, 1686.
2.   Voltaire, 'Physicians', *Philosophical Dictionary*.
3.   René Descartes, *Discourse on Method*, (Intro. A. D. Lindsay) Everyman's Library, J. M. Dent & Sons, 1912, p. VIII.
4.   Hall, *René Descartes; Treatise of Man*, cited in Harris L. Coulter, *Divided Legacy*, vol. II, Washington, Wehawken Book Co., 1975, p. 123.
5.   Lindsay, op. cit., pp. XIV-XV.
6.   Albert Lemoine, *Le Vitalisme et L'Animisme de Stahl*, Paris, Baillière, 1864, p. 103.
7.   Blondin, *Oevres de Stahl*, vol II, pp. 711; cited in Harris L. Coulter, *Divided Legacy*.
8.   Harris L. Coulter, op. cit., pp. 232–3.
9.   ibid., p. 238.
10. John Brown, *The Elements of Medicine*, 1804, pp. IXII–IXVII. Portsmouth, New Hampshire, Treadwell, 1804.
11. William Cullen, *Institutions of Medicine*, part I: Physiology, Edinburgh & Boston, Norman, 1788, p. 238.
12. Brown, op. cit., p. 116.
13. Wedekind, *Uber der Wertz der Heilkunde*, Darmstadt, 1812, p. 212.

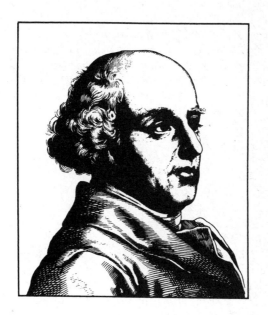

6 Hahnemann

Hahnemann, that rare combination of philosophy and learning, whose system must eventually bring about the ruin of the ordinary receipt-crammed heads, but is still little accepted by practitioners, and rather shunned than investigated.

Goethe, *Zerstr Blatter*, vol. II

Christian Frederich Samuel Hahnemann was born in 1755 in Meissen, in the Electorate of Saxony. His father was a painter and designer of porcelain in the famous Meissen porcelain factory. Hahnemann's childhood seems to have been much influenced by his father's example, and in later life he wrote of his father with great respect, as seen in this autobiographical fragment of 1791.

To act and live without pretence or show was his most noteworthy precept, which impressed me more by his example than by words. He was frequently present, though unobserved, when something good was to be accomplished. Should I not follow him? In his deeds he differentiated between noble and ignoble to so fine a degree of correctness and practical delicacy of feeling as to be highly creditable to him; in this he was also my teacher. His ideas on the first principles of creation, the dignity of mankind, and its lofty destiny, seemed consistent in every way with his mode of life. This was the foundation of my moral training.[1]

Richard Haehl, in his biography of Hahnemann, notes that his father brought his children up on the principles of Rousseau, ideas which were widely circulated amongst many cultured Europeans at that time. Hahnemann, himself, was a serious and dedicated student but, from time to time, thwarted by his father's straitened circumstances, he had to go to work. On one occasion, for example, he was apprenticed to a greengrocer. Fortunately, his outstanding intelligence and diligence were rewarded by the right to attend, free of charge, the Prince's School in Meissen. There, due to his already advanced knowledge of Greek and other languages, he helped to teach the other students. As a young man he dedicated himself to becoming an educated person; he often wrote that he had no childhood, as he constantly studied and worked.

Hahnemann's interest in science and medicine grew, and thus he left Meissen for Leipzig in 1775 to study medicine. Leipzig was a well-known medical university and yet it had no facilities for clinical training. Therefore, after two years of intensive studying, while supporting himself by teaching languages to other students and translating medical books from English to German, Hahnemann left for Vienna. There he studied with Dr Joseph Von Quarin who was the Royal Physician and could provide Hahnemann with the clinical teaching he so desperately wanted. He was, however, only able to remain there for nine months due to lack of funds. Von Quarin, recognizing his worth, found him a post as librarian to the Governor of Transylvania. After two years of cataloguing the Governor's library and continuing his language studies, Hahnemann enrolled at the University of Erlangen to complete his medical studies and there he received his degree in 1779.

For many years Hahnemann moved from place to place setting up practice (between 1782 and 1805 he moved seventeen times). Gradually, he became disillusioned with late eighteenth-century medical doctrines. Like Paracelsus and Van Helmont before him, he retired from practice between 1782–96, to search for answers to help him formulate a new approach to medicine. During those years he employed himself doing translations, writings and more chemical research.

At that time bloodletting was still very much in use, a method which Hahnemann violently opposed. Medical practice was, in general, still dominated by Cullen and Brown; also influential were the views of the German 'Natural Philosophers'

– to which Hahnemann was also opposed. Complex prescriptions, containing up to eight to ten drugs, were in daily use, as well as 'Magistral formulas', mixtures composed by 'authorities', which were remedies for various diseases, kept by the apothecaries as made-up medicines.

By 1796 Hahnemann had written the first important statement on the early formulation of homoeopathy; this was the 'Essay on a New Principle for Ascertaining the Curative Powers of Drugs, with a Few Glances at Those Hitherto Employed'. This was published in Hufeland's widely read *Journal der practischen Arzneykunde*.[2]

As already mentioned in chapter one, in this important essay Hahnemann put forward the idea that the most useful way in which to discover the full and exact curative powers of all medicines was to 'prove' them on healthy human beings.

Hahnemann was adamantly convinced that no method had yet been found to correctly understand the action of medicines. All other methods were haphazard as far as he was concerned, whether they chemically analysed a substance, tried them out on animals or in mixtures of blood, or tested them on the sick. He concluded that the only way to truly understand the action of a medicine was to carefully note every reaction and symptom created in a healthy human being when given that medicine. That is what he called a 'proving'. The observation of many individuals was necessary in order to create a full proving, and all symptoms, including mental and emotional, were recorded.

It was with the experiments that he made on himself with Cinchona bark, in 1790, while translating Cullen's *Materia Medica*[3], that Hahnemann had the kernel of the following idea: that the action a medicine had on a healthy person would prove curative on a sick person presenting those symtoms. Cullen had advocated Peruvian bark (Cinchona bark) as a specific for intermittent fever, by saying that its action was due to the tonic effect on the stomach caused by its bitter and astringent qualities. Hahnemann attacked this idea vigorously and experimented on himself to discover the actual reasons why Cinchona bark could cure intermittent fever. He discovered that, by taking doses of Cinchona bark, he himself produced all the symptoms of intermittent fever.

He wrote of this experiment:

> I took, for several days, as an experiment, four drams of good china [Cinchona bark] twice daily. My feet and finger tips, etc. at first became cold; I became languid and drowsy; then my heart began to palpitate; my pulse became hard and quick; and intolerable anxiety and trembling (but without a rigor); prostration in all the limbs; then pulsation in the head, redness of the cheeks, thirst; briefly, all the symptoms usually associated with intermittent fever appeared in succession, yet without actual rigor. To sum up: all those symptoms which to me are typical of intermittent fever, as the stupefaction of the senses, a kind of rigidity of all joints, but above all the numb disagreeable sensation which seems to have its seat in the periosteum over all the bones of the body – all made their appearance. This paroxysm lasted from two to three hours every time and recurred when I repeated the dose and not otherwise. I discontinued the medicine, and I was once more in good health.[4]

What proved important about this discovery for Hahnemann was that it showed him that one fever would cure another fever by the similarity between them. On this he said, 'Peruvian bark, which is used as a remedy for intermittent fever, acts because it can produce symptoms similar to those of intermittent fever in healthy people.'[5]

From this observation and induction ensued the important principle which Hahnemann called the 'Law of Similars'. It now became crucial to know the action of all medicines; therefore, accurate provings became very important. It is worth restating how Hahnemann presented this idea in the 1796 'Essay'. Every powerful medicinal substance produces in the human body a kind of peculiar disease; the more powerful the medicine, the more peculiar, marked, and violent the disease. We should imitate nature which sometimes cures a chronic disease by superadding another, and employ in the (especially chronic) disease we wish to cure, that medicine which is able to produce another very similar artificial disease, and the former will be cured; *similia similibus*.[6]

On provings, he says in the 'Essay': 'A complete collection of such observations, with remarks on the degree of reliance to be placed on their reporters would, if I mistake not, be the foundation stone of a *materia medica*, the sacred book of its revelation.'[7] He then expands further:

> We only require to know, on the one hand, the diseases of the human frame accurately in their essential characteristics, and their accidental complications, and, on the other hand, the pure effect of drugs, that is, the essential characteristics of the specific artificial disease they usually excite, together with the accidental symptoms caused by difference of dose, form etc., and by choosing a remedy for a given natural disease that is capable of producing a very similar artificial disease we shall be able to cure the most obstinate diseases.'[8]

Thus, the principle of the 'Law of Similars' became the foundation of homoeopathic practice from then onwards. (*refer to *Notes* at end of chapter 6)

Hahnemann knew there was virtually no knowledge of the effects of medicines on the healthy; he therefore carried out extensive series of provings throughout his lifetime, with the willing assistance of colleagues and students. These amounted to the provings of ninety-nine substances. More than 600 were added to the homoeopathic *Pharmacopoeia* by the end of the nineteenth century. Hahnemann's provings were presented in his *Fragmenta de Viribus Medicamentorum Positivis* (1805), containing his initial provings on himself and his family, and the *Materia Medica Pura* (1811–21), which contained the remainder.

As he was to state in his *Organon of Medicine*:

> There is . . . no other possible way in which the peculiar effects of medicine on the health of individuals can be accurately ascertained. There is no sure, no more natural way of accomplishing this object, than to administer the several medicines experimentally, in moderate doses, to *healthy* persons, in order to ascertain what changes, symptoms, and signs of their influence each individually produces on the health of the body and of the mind.[9]

In 1805 Hahnemann wrote a long article called 'The Medicine of Experience', in which he went into far more detail than in the earlier 'Essay', as to how to put these new methods of cure into practice. One point which he makes very clearly is the necessity of using only one single remedy at a time in the treatment of a given case. He says,

> If we wish to perceive clearly what the remedy effects in a disease, and what still remains to be done, we must only give one single simple substance at a time. Every addition of a second or a third only deranges the object we have in view. . . . It is . . . never necessary to administer more than one single simple medicinal substance at once, if it has been chosen appropriately to the case of the disease.[10]

Hahnemann was adamantly against the use of large mixtures of medicines, as was the common practice of the day. He had previously objected to the compounding of prescriptions because the effects of compounds in disease could not be known precisely. He observed that there was no methodical way of knowing what medicine was providing which effect. As he said elsewhere in a critique of compound prescription:

> Does it not occur to you that two dynamic agencies together can never effect that which each individually might, administered at different times? Do you not see that a middle effect must take place, which is not to be foreseen *a priori*? The heights of parempiricism are reached by prescribing multi-constituted prescriptions – perhaps many times a day. . . . It is as though one should throw blindfold a handfull of balls of various kinds upon an unknown billiard table with cushions of various angles, and should pretend to decide beforehand what effect they would all conjointly produce.[11]

This important concept of utilizing only one single, simple medicinal substance, became, and has remained, a basic tenet of homoeopathic practice.

The essay, 'The Medicine of Experience' was the forerunner of Hahnemann's definitive theoretical work, *Organon of the*

Rational Art of Healing, later to be called *Organon of the Healing Art*. The *Organon* was first published in 1810 while Hahnemann was still living in Torgau, and four successive editions were published during his lifetime, each edition expanded and altered.

He completed a sixth edition of the *Organon* by the end of his life, but this was not published until 1921. It is in this important work that the major elements of the homoeopathic method are explained in 294 numbered paragraphs; in this work Hahnemann first used the word homoeopathy. Throughout the *Organon*, he discusses the role of the 'vital force' in illness, health and cure, as well as outlining all the details of the homoeopathic method; the need for an exact procedure for doing provings; the smallness of dosage and the potentizing of remedies and their administration. Crucial to the *Organon* is the theory of the 'dynamis' in medicine and detailed information on the nature of the increase of strength by dilution, trituration and succussion of remedies.

The vital force is a most important concept to understand in homoeopathy. Hahnemann says of the vital force early in the *Organon*:

> In the healthy condition of man, the spiritual vital force, the dynamis that animates the material body, rules with unbounded sway, and retains all the parts of the organism in admirable, harmonious, vital operation, as regards both sensations and functions, so that our indwelling, reason-gifted mind can fully employ this living, healthy instrument for the higher purpose of existence . . . The material organization, without the vital force, is capable of no sensation, and performs all the functions of life solely by means of the immaterial being (the vital force) which animates the material organism in health and in disease.[12]

Thus, the vital force is deranged by the morbific agents of illness, and the

> morbidly affected vital force alone that produces diseases, so that the morbid phenomena perceptible to our senses express at the same time all the internal change, that is to say, the whole

morbid derangement of the internal dynamis; in a word, they reveal the whole disease; consequently, also, the disappearance under treatment of all the morbid phenomena and all of the morbid alterations that differ from the healthy vital operations, certainly affects and necessarily implies the restoration of the integrity of the vital force and, therefore, the recovered health of the whole organism.[13]

However, Hahnemann points out that the disturbed vital force cannot overcome this disturbance by itself; rather, it needs the aid of the correctly chosen remedy to do so.

The vital force was given to us to sustain our life in harmony as long as we are healthy, not to heal itself when diseased....
When afflicted by disease agents, our vital force can express its untunement only through disturbances in the normal functions of the organism and through pain, whereby it calls for the help of a wise physician.[14]

He amplifies this further in later writings, to show the reaction of the vital force and its role in the curative process: 'By giving a remedy which resembles the disease the instinctive vital force is compelled to increase its vital energy until it becomes stronger than the disease which, in turn, is vanquished.'[15]
And as stated more fully in the *Organon:*

So in homoeopathic cure this vital principle, which has been dynamically untuned by natural disease, is *taken over* by a similar and somewhat stronger artificial disease, through the administration of a potentized medicine that has been accurately chosen for the similarity of its symptoms.
Consequently the (weaker) natural dynamic disease is extinguished and disappears; from then on it no longer exists for the vital principle, which is controlled and occupied only by the stronger artificial disease; this in turn presently wanes, so that the patient is left free and cured. Thus delivered, the *dynamis* can again maintain the organism in health.[16]

While using and experimenting with similar medical agents Hahnemann observed that, if substantial amounts were

90

administered according to the law of similars, severe aggravation of the symptoms occurred. Thus he reduced the dosage to smaller and smaller amounts, eventually formulating his methods of dilution, trituration and succussion to create the smallest and more active doses. In the earlier years of his practice he had used doses comparable to his colleagues. He then reduced them and, by 1799, announced the principle of the infinitesimal dose. He justified this use of infinitesimal doses by experience.

> Has perchance Nature given us a law that we regard a scruple or a grain as the smallest and most suitable dose of all medicines – even of the most powerful? Has she not put knowledge and means into our hands so that we can arrange the more powerful and most powerful substances into smaller and smaller doses, some of them to a tenth of a grain, the more powerful to a hundredth or a thousandth of a grain, the highly powerful ones to a millionth, billionth, or even to a trillionth, quadrillionth and quintillianth of a grain? ...[17]

Hahnemann says of this process in the *Organon*:

> For its own special purpose and by its own special procedure, never tried before my time, homoeopathy develops the inner, spirit-like medicinal powers of crude substance to a degree hitherto unheard of and makes all of them exceedingly, even immeasurably, penetrating, active, and effective, even those that in the crude state do not have the slightest medicinal effect on the human organism.
>
> This remarkable transformation of the properties of natural bodies through the mechanical action of trituration and succussion on their tiniest particles (which particles are diffused in an inert dry or liquid substance) develops the latent *dynamic* powers previously imperceptible and as it were lying hidden asleep in them. These powers electively affect the vital principle of animal life. This process is called *dynamization* or *potentization* (development of medicinal power), and it creates what we call dynamization or potencies of different degrees.[18]

In *Divided Legacy* Harris Coulter describes the technique:

Hahnemann's technique was to mix one part of the medicine with 99 parts of milk sugar (if the medicine was dry) or 99 parts of alcohol (if the medicine was liquid) and then triturate it (if dry) or shake it (if liquid) for some time until the mass was uniformly mixed. This formed the 'first centesimal dilution' (if the ratio of medicinal substance to vehicle was 1:9, this was the 'first decimal dilution'). When one part of this dilution was thereupon mixed with another 99 parts of milk sugar or alcohol, and again triturated or succussed, the 'second centesimal dilution' was produced.[19]

In this process of potentization Hahnemann discovered that some substances, usually considered inert, would develop medicinal powers once triturated. Such substances as gold, silver, silica, ordinary salt, charcoal and Lycopodium (club moss) were amongst these. This also was the case with certain curative herbs. Hahnemann insisted that the remedies be prepared from fresh plants and, in this way, plants which had been considered ineffective by the old school of medicine, because they lost their medicinal value when dry, proved very effective when used by Hahnemann's method. These plants included Pulsatilla, Rhus Toxicodendron, Bryonia and many others.

Due to the minimalizing of dose and the process of dynamization, Hahnemann was able to make systematic use of poisons as medicines. By that process poisons can be carefully considered for their curative powers and, once diluted, do not have a 'poisonous effect'; on the contrary, a powerful, curative effect emerges. On this point Hahnemann comments:

Why should we reject after the manner of the childish and superstitious common folk those treasures of therapeutic value, which we really lack and which lie hidden in these potent substances? Why do we thrust them wantonly from us in our purist affection and ill conceived delicacy, when we could reduce them all by solution, dilution, and small administration to harmless efficiency, and so meet our requirements?[20]

Of course, when provings were done of poisons they were

done in dilution. Many poisons were transformed by the process of potentization and entered into the homoeopathic Pharmacopoeia; these included belladonna, strychnine, aconite, viper poison, various spider and snake poisons. They are still of great value in the homoeopathic *Pharmacopoeia* today.†

Paracelsus had seen this same inherent value in poisons when he said, 'Why then should poison be neglected and despised, if we consider not the poison but the curative virtue?'[21]

Hahnemann observed and maintained that, by this process of dilution, succussion and trituration, each successive 'potency' increased in its medicinal power. Thus, therapeutic action of a medicine increases with progressive dilution, so that, for instance, the second centesimal potency is more powerful than the first, and the tenth or thirtieth centesimals are more powerful still. He comments on this point:

> By the *succession* and *trituration*, there ensues not only the most intimate mixture, but at the same time – and this is the most important circumstance – there ensues such a great, and hitherto unknown and undreamt of change, by the development and liberation of the dynamic powers of the medicinal substance so treated, as to excite astonishment.[21]

At the time that Hahnemann was evolving and using this theory and practice of potency, considerable controversy was engendered by it, mainly (but not always) from outside the ranks of faithful homoeopaths. This was largely due to the fact that the Avogadro limit is reached at the 12th centesimal or 24th decimal dilution. The Avogadro limit is the point at which it is statistically improbable that the original medicinal substance will remain in the dilution. Hahnemann remained adamant about this method of potentizing remedies and continued to refine it until the end of his life.

Hahnemann's methods for making the remedies were so exacting that he made most of them himself, not trusting the apothecaries of his time. He insisted that homoeopathic physicians both make and dispense their own remedies. The pharmacists accused Hahnemann of 'entrenching upon their privileges by the dispensing of medicines'[22] and they brought the issue to court in 1820.

At that time Hahnemann had already had great therapeutic success with his new medical method. His reputation as a successful physician aroused the jealousy of his colleagues in Leipzig. When preparing a statement by which to defend himself in court, Hahnemann wrote:

The method of healing which I use for my patients is quite different from that of other doctors and consequently is not, like theirs, linked up with the work of the apothecary and to a certain extent dependent on him. The privilege of the apothecaries is limited to the dispensing of compound medicines, for which weight, price, etc. is prescribed for them. I, too, use remedies from nature, but they are only simple drugs. I must therefore deny entrenchment upon the privileges of the apothecaries by my own dispensing. Besides, I require my remedies only for my patients, not for sale to other people.[23]

A judgement, however, was made in favour of the apothecaries and ruled that Hahnemann was no longer allowed to distribute or dispense any medicines. Thus, once again, Hahnemann moved home, this time to the principality of the Duke of Anhalt-Koethen, where he remained from 1821–35. There he was allowed to both prepare and dispense his own medicines.

While in Koethen, Hahnemann published the third, fourth and fifth edition of the *Organon*, and also a second and third edition of the *Materia Medica Pura*. He also wrote on his new discoveries about the cause of chronic disease, set forth in *The Chronic Diseases* in five volumes.[24] He found, after several decades of treating patients with homoeopathic remedies, that certain cures were only temporary. After much thought, and looking at the possibility that not enough remedies had been proved, he concluded that there must be an underlying, inherited, chronic disease behind many cases.

He called these underlying chronic diseases 'miasms', and delineated the existence of three principal miasms. These were psora, syphilis and sycosis (gonorrhoea). He stated that all chronic diseases were caused by one of these three miasms. The word 'miasm' derives from the Greek and means taint or contamination. Hahnemann observed that the miasm, psora, accounted for seven eighths of all chronic disease. Psora was the oldest of the miasms and had manifested over the centuries as different diseases: leprosy in the Middle Ages, through various forms of erysipelas to the less virulent scabies. Syphilis and gonorrhoea had appeared in the sixteenth century, took root in the populations of Europe and were then passed on from generation to generation.

In *The Chronic Diseases* Hahnemann enumerated the symptoms of several new remedies, relating these remedies to the specific miasms to which they were connected. Many of the medicines introduced in *The Chronic Diseases* were destined to become very important in the practice of homoeopathy. As had been the case with the theory of potency, however, the new ideas on chronic disease provoked much discussion and controversy.

The main principle that Hahnemann observed was that, if the underlying chronic disease was tackled correctly, subsequent acute illnesses, no longer being complicated by the chronic one, were far easier to treat with success.

While in Koethen his wife died in 1830. For several years subsequently Hahnemann lived in near isolation. In 1835 he married again, however, to the thirty-five-year old, well born and beautiful Melanie d'Hervilly-Gohier. Soon after that he moved with her to Paris where he rapidly acquired a flourishing practice. He was already eighty years of age when he made this last move. Homoeopathy was, by this time, established in Paris and he was made welcome there although, as always, he remained a controversial figure. Melanie assisted him with his practice, studied with him and became a practitioner herself. These were the years in which Hahnemann wrote the sixth edition of the *Organon* which he completed before his death at eighty-eight, in 1843.

Hahnemann had led a long and industrious life, beleaguered at times by difficulties and controversy. As one of the great pioneers of medicine, however, he created a rich and lasting medical method. The story of the developments in homoeopathy throughout the latter part of the nineteenth century until today is a long and complex one, ever moving towards deeper and clearer understanding of the principles laid down by him.

We have seen some of the complexities of medical development from Paracelsus to Hahnemann, as ideas have interwoven with each other and created new syntheses. Out of this background came Hahnemann's unique and lasting medical system.

What is important is that homoeopathy is a system of medicine that can approach disease in its totality, encompassing the mental, emotional and physical, as well as the spiritual aspects of each individual. This system of medicine has spread around the world and is in great demand today.

As Hahnemann so clearly stated in the *Organon*:

All diseases are, in fact, diseases of the whole organism: no external malady... can arise, persist, or even grow worse without ... the cooperation of the whole organism, which must consequently be in a diseased state. It could not make its appearance at all without the consent of the whole of the rest of health, and without the participation of the rest of the living whole (of the vital force that pervades all the other sensitive and irritable parts of the organism); indeed, it is impossible to conceive its production without the instrumentality of the organism connected together to form an indivisible whole in sensations and functions.[26]

Underlying this very clear concept is Hahnemann's initial aim, stated at the beginning of the *Organon*: 'The highest ideal of therapy is to restore health rapidly, gently, permanently; to remove and destroy the whole disease in the shortest, surest, least harmful way, according to clearly comprehensible principles.'[27]

POSTSCRIPT TO CHAPTER 6

The Homoepathic model of treatment and cure, is in fact so unique as a totality, that it is most important to understand the possible precursors of these ideas, whilst seeing the timing of each progression of medical ideas clearly in their historical context. Its philosophy, structure and methodology are all united; integrated theory and practice.

Despite Hahnemann's scholarship and extensive writings, he was not one to often cite past medical authorites or ideas, save to criticize thinkers he felt were harmful or misleading. Occassionally he mentions, in a footnote, the odd contemporary or recent precursor whose work he praises. Nor does he mention in his writings many of his other philosophical interests or influences outside the medical field. For the historian this poses the problem of supposition, hypothesis or interpretation. We do know that in an early stage of his medical career he was given an entry to a Masonic Lodge. Little or nothing exists in documentation to enlighten us as to his actual interests, affiliation or influences therein. That he had an enormous respect for a 'divine source' in the world does come through his writings, but no apparent religion symbolism is there, no reference to any form or structure that can be pinned down.

That he was versed in some form of esoteric thought does seem most probable, again witnessed as inference in various ideas and writings. The Masonic element in Germany at that time would have been a development from the earlier Rosicrucian imput, although no doubt very different to the seventeenth century original formation. Men of science and medicine had, since the time of the formation of the 'societies', chosen these groups as a way to promote knowledge as well as supporting each other in the pursuit of that knowledge. As the history of Freemasonry is an enormous subject and very complex in itself, one does not want to make too much of this aspect of Hahnemann's life, mainly as it is so undocumented. However, influences must have existed in his Life leading him to his specific ideas, not solely from the medical lore of his day.

His 'spirit-like', dynamis, resonates of Stahl's 'anima' and vital force, of Van Helmont's and Paracelsus's 'archeus', and yet he brought his concept of the vital force into very clear focus by discovering a medicinal equivalent to match this 'invisible' but all pervasive kernel of each human being. This was Hahnemann's genius, to bring into play a medicinal force as subtle and equally as forceful as the complexity of the ever changing, idiosyncratic nature of individual human beings. A truly exact science, which covers man's inheritance, frailties, inner strength, psyche and soma. Hahnemann continued right up until his death to refine his methods and concepts, ever aiming at cure through the gentlest and most accurate of means. The task of continuing the research and refinement has been left to successive generations of Homoeopaths. From our perspective there is still always a great deal to learn from his work.

Notes – Chapter 6

1. Richard Haehl, *Samuel Hahnemann, His Life and Work*, London, Homoeopathic Publishing Co., 1922, p. 10.
2. Hufeland, *Journal der practischen Arzneykunde*, vol. II, part III, 1796.
3. William Cullen, *Abhandlung ueber die Materia Medica*, Leipzig, im Schwickersten Verlag, 1790, Vol. II, pp. 108–9.
4. Haehl, op. cit., p. 37.
5. Samuel Hahnemann, *Lesser Writings*, London, W. Headland, 1851, pp. 311–12.
6. ibid., p. 311.
7. ibid., p. 312.
8. Hahnemann, *Organon of the Rational Art of Healing* (trans. R.E. Dudgeon and W. Boericke), Dresden, Arnold, 1810, para. 108.
   This work went through five editions in Hanemann's lifetime, the sixth published in 1921; all references fifth and sixth edition unless otherwise stated.
9. Hahnemann, *Lesser Writings*, London, W. Headland, 1851, p. 534.
10. ibid., pp. 346–49.
11. Hahnemann, *Organon*, paras 9, 10.
12. ibid., para. 12.
13. ibid., (Victor Gollancz, 1983, London, J. Kunzli et al.), para. 22, footnote (a).
14. Hahnemann, *The Chronic Diseases, Their Peculiar Nature and Their Homoeopathic Cure* (trans. L. H. Tafel), Philadelphia, Boericke and Tafel, 1904.
15. Hahnemann, *Organon* (trans. J. Kunzli et al.), London, Victor Gollanz, 1983, para. 29.
16. Haehl, op. cit., vol. I, p. 314.
17. Hahnemann, *Organon* (trans. J. Kunzli et al), London, Victor Gollancz, 1983, para. 269.
18. Harris L. Coulter, *Divided Legacy*, Washington, Wehawken Book Co., 1977, vol. II, p. 401.
19. Haehl, op. cit., vol. I, p. 76.

20. Alan Debus, *The English Paracelsians,* London, Oldbourne, 1965.
21. Hahnemann, *Lesser Writings*, London, W. Headland, 1851, pp. 817–18.
22. Haehl, op. cit., vol. I, p. 108.
23. ibid.
24. Hahnemann, *The Chronic Diseases, Their Peculiar Nature and Their Homoeopathic Cure* (trans. L. H. Tafel), Philadelphia, Boericke and Tafel, 1904, vol. IV, p.4.
25. Hahnemann, (trans. J. Kunzli et al.,) London, Victor Gollancz, 1983, para. 189.
26. ibid., para. 2.

Additional Notes

*p. 86 The concept and method of 'proving' drugs became the basis of the Homoeopathic *materia medica*, and still is to this day. Perhaps this is one of the greatest contributions Hahnemann made to medicine. For, with the 'proving' of drugs, Hahnemann made a crucial and innovative contribution to the history of medicine. Clearly the system is a total system of cure, however, in terms of the progression of ideas we have examined, the 'proving' is what separates Hahnemann from the past, and brings his idea forward to the formation of a total system.

†p. 92 Hahnemann, like Paracelsus, and possibly due to him, made metals and minerals truly available as medicinal agents; he not only saw great value in poisons, but also in the great metals, many of which were being discovered at that point in time by exploring minerologists. Gold and silver, only two amongst the many important remedies made from metals, were 'proved' systematically by Hahnemann and his students. Many other important metals and minerals have been 'proved' since, and take an important place in the Homoeopathic materia medica. These of course differed from Paracelsus's mineral and metal remedies, in that they were Homoepathically potentized, thus reaching even greater depths of curative action.

Bibliography

Ameke, W., *History of Homoeopathy*, London, Gould, 1885.

Bacon, F., *The Advancement of Learning*, New York, Willey Book Co. 1900.

Bettoli, U. A., *Dissertazione critico-Medico sul Sistema del Sig. Stahl,* 1791.

Boorstin, D. J., *The Discoverers*, New York, Vintage Books, 1985.

Bradford, T. L., *The Life and Letters of Samuel Hahnemann*, 1895 (reprinted New Dehli, B. Jain Publishers 1986).

Clark, G. N., *The Seventeenth Century*, Clarendon Press, 1929 (reprinted Oxford University Press, 1960.

Coulter, H. L., *Divided Legacy. A History of the Schism in Medical Thought*, vol I: *The Patterns Emerge: Hippocrates to Paracelsus*, 1975; vol. II: *Progress and Regress: J. B. Van Helmont to Claude Bernard*, Washington, Wehawken Book Co., 1977.

Dee, J., *Heptarchia mystica*, Aquarian Press, 1986.

Debus, A. G., *The Chemical Philosophy*, 2 Vols, New York, Science History Publications, 1977. *The English Paracelsians*, London, Oldbourne History of Science Library, 1965.

Descartes, R., *A Discourse on Method*, London, J. M. Dent & Sons, 1912.

Dudgeon, R. E., *Hahnemann, the Founder of Scientific Therapeutics*, 1882.

Eliade, M., *A History of Religious Ideas*, vol. 3, Chicago, University of Chicago Press, 1985.

French, P. J., *John Dee – the World of an Elizabethan Magus.* London, Routledge, Kegan & Paul, 1972.

Garrison, F. H., *An Introduction to the History of Medicine*, Philadelphia, Saunders.

Grossinger, R., *Planet Medicine, from Stone Age Shamanism to Post-Industrial Healing*, Boulder & London, Shambhala, 1982.

Haehl, R., *Samuel Hahnemann, His Life and Work*, 2 vols, London, Homoeopathic Publishing Co., 1922.

Hahnemann, Samuel, *The Chronic Diseases, Their Peculiar Nature and Their Homoeopathic Cure* (trans. L. H. Tafel), Philadelphia, Boericke and Tafel, 1904, (reprinted New Dehli, Jain Publishing Co., 1980.

Materia Medica Pura, 2 vols. (trans. R. E. Dudgeon), London, Homoeopathic Publishing Co., 1880, 1936 (reprinted Calcutta, M. Bhattacharyya and Co., 1952.

Hahnemann, Samuel, *Organon of the Rational Art of Healing* (trans. E. Dudgeon & W. Boericke), Dresden, Arnold, 1810 (reprinted Calcutta, Toy Publishing House, 1961) and *Organon of the Rational Art of Healing* (trans. J. Kunzli et al.), London, Victor Gollancz, 1983.

Hahnemann, Samuel, *Lesser Writings* collected and translated by R.E. Dudgeon, New York, Radde, 1852.

Hill, C., 'Newton and his Society', *The Annus Mirabilis of Sir Isaac Newton 1666–1966,* Cambridge Mass. & London, MIT Press, 1970.

Hobhouse, R. W., *Life of Christian Samuel Hahnemann,* London, C. W. Daniel Co., 1933.

Holmyard, E. J., *Makers of Chemistry,* O.U.P. 1931.

Jacobi, J. (ed.), *Selected Writings of Paracelsus*(trans. Norbert Guterman), Bollinger Series XXVIII, Princeton University Press, 1973).

Koestler, A., *The Sleepwalkers. A History of Man's Changing Vision of the Universe,* London, Pelican Books, 1968.

Kuhn, T. S., *The Structure of Scientific Revolutions,* University of Chicago Press, 1970.

Leeser, O., *The Contribution of Homoeopathy to the Development of Medicine,* London, Hippocrates Publishing Co., 1943.

Lemoine, A., *Le Vitalisme et l'animisme de Stahl,* Paris, Baillière, 1864.

Mason, S. F., *A History of the Sciences*, New York, Collier Books, 1962.

Metzger, H., *Newton, Stahl, Boerhaave et la Doctrine Chimique,* Paris, 1930.

Mitchell, G. R., *Homoeopathy: The First Authoritative Study of Its Place in Medicine Today,* London, W. H. Allen, 1975.

Pachter, H. M., *Paracelsus. Magic into Science,* New York, Henry Schuman, 1951.

Pagel, W., *Paracelsus, an Introduction to Philosophical Medicine in the Era of the Renaissance*, Basel, S. Karger, 1958.

Pagel, W., 'Paracelsus and the Neo-Platonic and Gnostic Tradition', London, *Ambix*, 8, 1960.

The Religious and Philosophical Aspects of Van Helmont's Science & Medicine, Baltimore, The Johns Hopkins Press, 1949.

*The Smiling Spleen. Paracelsianism• in Storm and Stress,*Basel, S. Karger, 1984.

'Van Helmont's Concept of Disease – To be or not to be? The Influence of Paracelsus', *Bulletin of the History of Medicine,* vol. XLVI, no. 5, Sept.–Oct. 1972.

Paracelsus Werke (ed. Karl Sudhoff), 5 vols., Basel, Schwabe & Co., 1965.

Ponce, C., *Papers towards a Radical Metaphysics – Alchemy,* Berkeley, North Atlantic Books, 1983.

Rattansi, P. M., *Paracelsus and the Puritan Revolution, Ambix,* vol. XI, no. 1, 1963.

Read, J., *Prelude to Chemistry,* London, G. Bell and Son, 1936.

Risse, G. B., '*Kant, Schilling, and the Early Search for a Philosophical "Science" of Medicine in Germany*', *Journal of the History of Medicine and Allied Sciences,* vol. XXVII, no. 2, New Haven, Conn., 1972.

Sherlock, T. P., 'The Chemical Work of Paracelsus', London, *Ambix*, 3, 1948.

Shumaker, W., *The Occult Sciences in the Renaissance,* Berkeley, Los Angeles, London, University of California Press, 1972.

Steiner, R., *Eleven European Mystics,* New York, Rudolf Steiner Publications, 1971.

Sudhoff, K. (ed.), *Paracelsus Werke,* 15 vols., Munich & Berlin, Druct und Verlag von R. Oldenburg, 1922–33.

Thorndyke, L., *History of Magic and Experimental Science,* vols. V–VIII, New York, Columbia University Press, 1958.

Van Helmont, J. B., *Ortus Medicinae,* 1648.

Oriatrike, or Physick Refined, London, 1662.

Waite, A. E., (trans.), *The Hermetic and Alchemical Writings of Paracelsus,* 2 vols, (reprinted Berkeley 1874, Shambhala, 1976).

Weir, J., *The Science and Art of Homoeopathy,* vol. II, 9th Quinquennial International Homoeopathic Congress, 1927.

Yates, F., *The Rosicrucian Enlightenment,* London, Paladin, 1975.

Index

Advancement of Learning, The (Bacon) 60-1
Agrippa, Cornelius 14, 61
alchemy 14, 18, 20-1, 49, 55-6, 60, 61, 62, 63
Alchemy, the Third Column of Medicine (Paracelsus) 20-1
allopathic medicine 3-4
Andrae, J.V. 66
Anima Sensitiva 74-6
arcana 21, 24, 25, 45
archeus 22, 39-41, 42, 44
Archidoxies (Paracelsus) 27
Aristotle/Aristotelians 13, 15, 19, 37, 60, 73
Ashmole, Elias 62-63
astrology 61
Atalanta Fugiens (Maier) 58
Avicenna 15, 28

Bacon, Francis 47, 50, 55, 59-62, 71
Baglivi 75, 76
Barthez, Paul-Joseph 77
Boerhaave, Hermann 74-5
Bohme, Jakob 63
Bordeu, Theophile 77
Boyle, Robert 72
Brown, John 78-9, 80-1
Bruno, Giordano 59

Cabalistic tradition 14, 47, 56, 61
Calvin, John 37
Catholicism 28, 51, 54, 71
Christianity 28, 44, 55, 57, 69
Chronic Diseases, The (Hahnemann) 93-4
Cinchona bark 8, 84-5
Columbo, Realdo 37
Comenius 66
Concerning the Fabric of the Human Body (Vesalius) 37
Copernicus, Nicolas 2, 36
Coulter, Harris 41, 75, 91
Cullen, William 78-9, 84-5

Das Zweite Buch der Grossen Wundarznei (Paracelsus) 14
Debus, Alan 17, 19, 33
Dee, John 50, 51-4, 56, 57, 59, 60, 63, 66
De Materia Verae Medicinae Philosophorum Priscorum (Duchesne) 35
Descartes, René 71-3
Discourse on Method (Descartes) 70
Divided Legacy (Coulter) 77, 91
Duchesne, Joseph 34-5
dynamization 90-1

Einstein, Albert 2, 47
Elizabeth I 53
Eliade, Mircea 65
English Paracelsians, The (Debus) 17–18, 19
ens 26–7
Erasistratos 15
'Essay on a New Principle for Ascertaining the Curative Power(s) of Drugs' (Hahnemann) 5–8, 84, 85–6, 87

Febrium Doctrina Inaudita (Van Helmont) 44
Ficino, Marsilio 52, 54, 58
Fludd, Robert 34, 50, 51, 56, 58, 62, 66
Fontenelle, Bernard le Bovyer de 68
Fragmenta de Viribus Medicamentorum Positivis (Hahnemann) 86
Francis Bacon, From Magic to Science (Rossi) 61
Frederick William I of Prussia 75
French, Peter 51
Fuggers 17, 23

Galen/Galenist medicine 13, 15, 16, 19, 20, 28, 33, 34, 35, 36, 37, 38, 39, 42, 43
Galilei, Galileo 36, 63, 72
Goethe, J.W. von 83

Hahnemann, Christian Frederich Samuel 1–13, 29, 30, 70, 78, 80, 83*ff*
Haehl, Richard 12, 83
Harvey, William 37–8, 70

Helmont, Franciscus Mercurius Van 44–5
Helmont, Jan Baptista Van 33, 38–46, 51, 84
Henry IV 35–6
Hermes Trismegistus 27
Hermetic school 14, 20, 21, 27, 41, 47, 50, 51, 53, 54, 58, 59, 60, 61, 62, 65
Hervilly-Gohier, Melanie d' 94
Hill, Christopher 64
Hippocrates 11, 13, 15, 41, 76
History of Religious Ideas, A (Eliade) 65
Hoffman, C.L. 79
Hoffman, Friedrich 74, 79
Hufeland, Christoph Wilhelm 4
humours 15–16, 19

iatrochemists 19, 23, 33–47
infinitesimal dose 90–1
Islamic alchemy 18

James I 36, 53, 60
Jenner, Edward 8
Jennis, Lucas 58
Journal der practischen Arzneykunde (Hufeland) 84
Judaism 14
Jung, Carl Gustav 30

Kepler, Johann 36, 63
Koestler, Arthur 65
Kuhn, Thomas S. 2, 3

Labrinthus Medicorum Errantium vom Irrgang der Arzte (Paracelsus) 24
Lavoisier, Antoine Laurent 8
'Law of Similars' 85, 86

Lesser Writings (Hahnemann) 4–5
'like cures like' 8
Lutheranism 51

Maier, Michael 50, 51, 56, 58–9
Magia 56, 61
Magna Instauratio 60
Materia Medica Pura (Cullen, Hahnemann) 8, 85, 87, 94
Mayerne, Theodore Turquet de 35–6
'Medicine of Experience, The' Hahnemann) 88–9
Mirandola, Pico della 52, 57
Monas Hieroglyphica (Dee) 52–3
Mysterium Magnum 22

neo-Platonists 14, 20, 29, 41, 42, 51, 52, 54, 59
New Atlantis, The (Bacon) 62
Newton, Sir Isaac 2, 47, 50, 55, 59, 62–4, 66, 73
'Newton and his Society' (Hill) 62*ff*
Novum Organum (Bacon) 59*ff*

On the Motion of the Heart and Blood (Harvey) 37
Opuscula Medica Inaudita (Van Helmont) 44, 45
Organon of Medicine (a.k.a. *Organon of the Rational Art of Healing; Organon of the Healing Art:* Hahnemann) 87*ff*
Oration on the Dignity of Man (Mirandola) 57
Oriatrike (Van Helmont) 41, 43, 46

Ortus Medicinae (Van Helmont) 45

Pagel, Walter 33, 46
Paracelsus/Paracelsians 11–30, 33, 34–5, 36, 37, 38, 39, 40, 41, 44, 45, 46, 49–50, 55, 56, 58, 59, 66, 84, 93*ff*
Paragranum (Paracelsus) 21
Petrarch 52
Pharmacopoeia 34, 36, 87, 93
Philosophia de Generationibus et Fructus Quartor Elementorum (Paracelsus) 19
Plurality of Words (Fontenelle) 68
potentization 91–3
Primerose, James 34
Principia (Newton) 62, 64
Promissa Autoris (Van Helmont) 38
Protestantism 51, 57
'proving' 8, 86
Pythagorean principles 51

Quarin, Joseph Von 84
Quercetanus 35

Rosicrucian Enlightenment, The (Yates) 47, 50, 55
Rosicrucianism 49–66
Rosie, Paolo 61
Rousseau, Jean Jacques 82
Royal Society of Medicine 9, 62
Rudolph II 56

Sauvages, François Bossier de la Croix de 76, 77
semina 40
Servetus, Michael 37

similia similibus 8, 9, 86–7
Sleepwalkers, The (Koestler) 65
Smiling Spleen, The (Pagel) 33
Stahl, George Ernest 73–7, 80
Stoics 16
Structure of Scientific Revolutions, The (Kuhn) 2
Sydenham, Thomas 76
sympathetic action 42

Theatrum Chemicum Britannicum Fama Fraternitatis (Ashmole) 49, 55, 63
Trithemius, Abbot of Sponheim 14

Twelve Gates into the City, The (Danciger) 13
Tymme, Thomas 35

Vesalius 36, 37
Voltaire, François 71

Weir, Sir John 9

Yates, Francis 47, 50, 55, 56, 61, 63

Zerstr Blatter (Goethe) 83